Final Evaluation Report for the TRICARE Senior Supplement Demonstration Program

Michael Schoenbaum
Katherine Harris
Gary Cecchine
Ana Suarez
Chris Horn
C. Ross Anthony

Prepared for the Office of the Secretary of Defense

National Defense Research Institute | RAND Health

RAND

The research described in this report was sponsored by the Office of the Secretary of Defense (OSD). The research was conducted jointly by RAND Health's Center for Military Health Policy Research and the Forces and Resources Policy Center of the National Defense Research Institute, a federally funded research and development center supported by the OSD, the Joint Staff, the unified commands, and the defense agencies. It was performed under contracts DASW01-95-C-0059 and DASW01-01-C-0004, "TRICARE Senior Supplement and Uniformed Services Family Health Plan Demonstration Evaluations," Michael Schoenbaum, Principal Investigator.

Library of Congress Cataloging-in-Publication Data

MR-1549 : final evaluation report for the TRICARE senior supplement demonstration
  program / Michael Schoenbaum ... [et al.].
     p. cm.
   ISBN 0-8330-3194-5
   1. Medicine, Military. 2. Retired military personnel—Medical care. 3. Military
dependents—Medical care. 4. Managed care plans (Medical care) I. Schoenbaum,
Michael.

RC971 .M723 2002
368.4'26'0086970973—dc21

                                                                    2002068116

Published 2002 by RAND
1700 Main Street, P.O. Box 2138, Santa Monica, CA 90407-2138
1200 South Hayes Street, Arlington, VA 22202-5050
201 North Craig Street, Suite 202, Pittsburgh, PA 15213-1516
RAND URL: http://www.rand.org/
To order RAND documents or to obtain additional information, contact Distribution
Services: Telephone: (310) 451-7002; Fax: (310) 451-6915; Email: order@rand.org

Preface

The TRICARE Senior Supplement Demonstration (TSSD) is a congressionally authorized program that offers certain Medicare-eligible military beneficiaries the option of enrolling in TRICARE as a supplement to Medicare. TSSD enrollment began in March 2000, and the program was scheduled to run through December 2002. However, the value of TSSD as a demonstration program was reduced by the passage of the 2001 National Defense Authorization Act, which provides for TRICARE for Life (TFL). TFL is a permanent national supplemental insurance benefit for Medicare-eligible military beneficiaries. TFL has been available as of October 2001 and has among the most comprehensive health insurance benefits in the United States. Because of TFL and other factors, the number of beneficiaries eligible for TSSD who opted to enroll in the program was very low. Within this context, we wrote this book to meet a congressional requirement for a report that evaluates TSSD and makes recommendations about its suitability as a permanent national program. Our evaluation includes consideration of how the Department of Defense's experience with TSSD would be relevant to the new TFL program. This book should interest defense health policymakers and individuals in health care benefits management in both the private and public health care sectors.

This book underscores the importance of providing clear and comprehensive information to beneficiaries regarding their health insurance benefits and illustrates the challenges of administering supplemental benefits and coordinating claims. In addition, we found that the temporary nature of TSSD, combined with uncertainty about whether enrollees would be able to reinstate private supplemental coverage if they dropped that coverage to join TSSD, is likely to result in reduced enrollment in the program. These factors, in turn, diminish the program's value as a potential model for providing supplemental health insurance benefits to Medicare-eligible military beneficiaries.

This work is sponsored by the Health Program Analysis and Evaluation Unit of TRICARE Management Activity under the Assistant Secretary of Defense for Health Affairs. The project is being carried out jointly by RAND Health's Center for Military Health Policy Research and the Forces and Resources Policy Center of the National Defense Research Institute (NDRI). NDRI is a federally funded research and development center sponsored by the Office of the Secretary of Defense, the Joint Staff, the unified commands, and the defense agencies.

Contents

Figures

..

Tables

Summary

The National Defense Authorization Act (NDAA) for fiscal year 1999 directed the Secretary of Defense to establish a demonstration program, called the TRICARE Senior Supplement Demonstration (TSSD), under which eligible beneficiaries would be permitted to enroll in the Department of Defense (DOD) TRICARE health insurance program as a supplement to Medicare. Congress directed the DoD to demonstrate TSSD in two geographic areas, with enrollment beginning in March 2000 and the program ending in December 2002. The DoD was required to submit a report to Congress by December 31, 2002, evaluating TSSD and making recommendations about its suitability as a permanent national program. The DoD selected RAND to perform this evaluation and address the issues identified by Congress. This document represents RAND's final evaluation report to the DoD.

Background on the TSSD Program and TRICARE for Life

Until October 1, 2001, when the TRICARE for Life (TFL)[1] program became available, Medicare-eligible military retirees and their Medicare-eligible dependents had only limited entitlement to military-sponsored health care. Historically, military retirees became ineligible for TRICARE at age 65 when they qualified for Medicare. Such beneficiaries were entitled to receive care in military treatment facilities (MTFs) on a space-available basis but could not use other DoD-sponsored health insurance benefits.

The 1999 NDAA (PL 105-261) included provisions for several alternative demonstration programs to provide supplemental health insurance benefits to Medicare-eligible military retirees. Section 722 authorized the DoD to implement the TSSD program. Under the TSSD, certain Medicare-eligible DoD beneficiaries were offered the opportunity to enroll in TRICARE as a supplement to Medicare and to receive prescription drug coverage through the National Mail Order Pharmacy (NMOP) and TRICARE civilian network pharmacies.

---

[1]TFL is a permanent national supplemental insurance benefit for Medicare-eligible military beneficiaries; it includes a comprehensive prescription drug benefit that was available as of April 2001.

Eligible beneficiaries could enroll in TSSD beginning in spring 2000, and the demonstration is scheduled to end December 31, 2002. TSSD is being conducted in and around Santa Clara County, California, and Cherokee County, Texas. An eligible beneficiary must reside in a defined area around these locations and must also be either a retiree of the Uniformed Services, a dependent of a Uniformed Services retiree, or the dependent survivor of a Uniformed Services retiree or member. Additionally, eligible beneficiaries are age 65 or over, are eligible for Medicare Part A, and are enrolled in Medicare Part B. Beneficiaries enrolled in TSSD are not eligible to receive care or pharmaceuticals from military health care facilities.

While the TSSD demonstration was under way, the U.S. Congress passed the 2001 National Defense Authorization Act, which authorized the TFL program. As of October 1, 2001, TFL provides TRICARE as supplemental health insurance for all Medicare-eligible military retirees who are enrolled in Medicare Part B. In general, TFL covers all cost-sharing for Medicare-covered services and standard TRICARE cost-sharing for services that are covered by TRICARE but not by Medicare. Because TFL is a permanent national program designed to address the same goals as TSSD addresses, TFL changed the policy context in which TSSD was taking place by preempting the possibility that the TRICARE Senior Supplement Demonstration program would be instituted in any permanent way.

Because of the introduction of TFL, and the fact that TSSD enrollment was very low, RAND and the DoD revised the evaluation plan for TSSD. The overall goal remained the same: to provide the information requested by Congress regarding the experience of the TSSD demonstration. Given the passage and subsequent implementation of TFL, we additionally considered ways in which the DoD's experience with TSSD would be relevant to TFL.

Research Methods

Our evaluation activities included interviews with TSSD program staff, collection and review of written materials about the program, focus groups that included TSSD enrollees and eligible beneficiaries, and a mail survey of TSSD enrollees and eligible beneficiaries.

Research Findings

TSSD enrollment was very low, in terms of both absolute numbers (approximately 350 enrollees out of 11,000) and in the fraction of eligible beneficiaries (slightly more than 3 percent). Married, higher-income, and relatively healthy beneficiaries were somewhat more likely to enroll than single, lower-income, and less-healthy beneficiaries, as were members of military retiree organizations and beneficiaries who retired as officers. Beneficiaries with employer-sponsored supplemental coverage prior to TSSD, or with Medicare health maintenance organization (HMO) coverage, were somewhat less likely to enroll than those without such sources of coverage.

We identified a number of factors that are likely to have inhibited enrollment in TSSD:

- Awareness of TSSD appeared to be low among eligible beneficiaries.

- Some beneficiaries confused TSSD with TRICARE Prime or, after its introduction, with TFL. The latter confusion was reinforced by the decision of the TRICARE Management Activity (TMA)[2] to stop publicizing TSSD due to difficulties in administering the benefit and in processing claims.

- Understanding of the TSSD benefit also appeared to be imperfect among beneficiaries who were aware of the program and even among enrollees themselves.

- TSSD beneficiaries had to receive care from TRICARE network providers in order to receive the maximum benefit, avoid liability for charges exceeding the Medicare reimbursement rates, and avoid the need to file paper claims.

- Finally, and perhaps most important, beneficiaries were uncertain about their rights to reinstate their prior, or other comparable, supplemental insurance coverage at the end of the demonstration period. This uncertainty seems understandable because in our view it is likely that beneficiaries did not have a statutory right to reinstatement (e.g., under the Balanced Budget Act of 1997).

Conclusions

The TSSD evaluation confirmed the importance of adequate health care decision support for beneficiaries. With TSSD—a demonstration program being conducted in two relatively confined geographic areas and with a clearly defined population of eligible beneficiaries—the DoD encountered difficulties educating eligible beneficiaries about the demonstration. This issue will be just as important for TFL, and our findings suggest that the DoD may face considerable challenges in communicating with TFL beneficiaries.

---

[2]TMA is an office within the Department of Defense with responsibility for overseeing the administration of health benefits to military dependents and retirees.

A second policy issue that applies to TSSD and TFL is the likely substitution of DoD-sponsored health insurance benefits for existing supplemental coverage. We found that TSSD beneficiaries with existing employer-sponsored coverage, in particular, were less likely to enroll in TSSD than those without employer-sponsored coverage, whereas those with prior private Medicare supplemental plans (commonly referred to as "Medigap" plans) were more likely to enroll than those without Medigap. In general, TFL has both more-generous benefits and lower out-of-pocket costs than TSSD or most other types of supplemental coverage. As a result, it seems likely that beneficiaries with current supplemental coverage, including employer-sponsored coverage, will drop such coverage in favor of TFL.

Overall, our results suggest that implementation of TSSD as a permanent national program would be feasible, although it is clearly unlikely to happen. Furthermore, a national program based on TSSD would have relatively high actuarial value for beneficiaries relative to private Medigap policies and many employer-sponsored supplemental plans (and relative to no supplemental insurance). A TSSD-based program also would have lower costs for the Department of Defense than would TFL due to the fact that TSSD retains modest cost-sharing for beneficiaries and a preferred-provider network structure. Any national implementation of TSSD, however, would require revision of the procedures for administering the benefit and processing claims.

Acknowledgments

We are grateful to Barbara Wynn and Jeanne Ringel for their review comments, Melissa Bradley for help with survey activities, Scott Ashwood for programming assistance, Terri Tanielian for outstanding administrative management, and Nancy DelFavero for editing of the final report. We are also grateful to the many people who participated in focus groups or agreed to be interviewed or surveyed for this project.

Acronyms

AFB	Air Force Base
BBA	Balanced Budget Act
BRAC	Base realignment and closure
CHAMPUS	Civilian Health and Medical Program of the Uniformed Services
DEERS	Defense Enrollment Eligibility Reporting System
DoD	Department of Defense
ESRD	End-stage renal disease
FEHBP	Federal Employee Health Benefit Program
FY	Fiscal year
HMO	Health maintenance organization
MTF	Military treatment facility
NDAA	National Defense Authorization Act
NMOP	National Mail Order Pharmacy
OMB	Office of Management and Budget
TMA	TRICARE Management Activity
TFL	TRICARE for Life
TROA	The Reserve Officers Association
TSSD	TRICARE Senior Supplement Demonstration
USPS	United States Postal Service
VA	Department of Veterans Affairs

1. Introduction

This document represents the final report of RAND's evaluation of the TRICARE
Senior Supplement Demonstration (TSSD), a congressionally authorized health
insurance program that offered certain Medicare-eligible military beneficiaries
the option of enrolling in the Department of Defense (DoD) TRICARE health
insurance program as a supplement to Medicare. TSSD enrollment began in
March 2000, and the program was scheduled to run through December 2002.

During the course of TSSD, the U.S. Congress enacted TRICARE for Life (TFL)[1]
with an accompanying pharmacy benefit as a permanent national program for
Medicare-eligible military beneficiaries. Therefore, TSSD clearly is not being
considered as a permanent national program. For this reason, and because TSSD
enrollment was very low (both in absolute terms and as a fraction of the eligible
population), the scope and nature of this evaluation were revised midway
through the project. Throughout this report, we focus on lessons from the TSSD
program that could help inform TFL implementation and administration and
other health policy issues for military retirees.

Policy Context of the TRICARE Senior Supplement Demonstration

Until October 2001, Medicare-eligible military retirees and their Medicare-eligible
dependents had only limited entitlement to military-sponsored health care. For
beneficiaries under age 65, the DoD provides medical care through the TRICARE
program, which consists of TRICARE Prime, Standard, and Extra. TRICARE
Prime is essentially a health maintenance organization (HMO); the provider
network consists primarily of military treatment facilities (MTFs) (the "direct
care" system), supplemented by care from designated civilian providers as
authorized (the "purchased care" system). The services operated about 465
military treatment facilities in 1999, representing 91 hospitals and 374 clinics
(U.S. General Accounting Office, 1999). TRICARE Standard and Extra both
essentially function as a preferred-provider organizations, with TRICARE Extra

---

[1]TFL is a permanent national supplemental insurance benefit for Medicare-eligible military
beneficiaries; it includes a comprehensive prescription drug benefit that was available as of April
2001.

representing the in-network benefit and TRICARE Standard the out-of-network benefit.

Since 1966, however, military retirees became ineligible for TRICARE at age 65 when they qualify for Medicare. Such beneficiaries were entitled to receive care in MTFs on a space-available basis but could not use other DoD-sponsored health insurance benefits.[2] Because Medicare benefits were generally less comprehensive and more expensive than TRICARE benefits, retirees and their advocacy groups believed, and argued in a series of court cases, that this policy violated a commitment that the DoD had made to provide military personnel with health insurance coverage for life.[3] The groups had lobbied Congress for years to honor this commitment.

Congress acted in a number of ways to address this issue. The 1999 National Defense Authorization Act (NDAA) (PL 105-261) included provisions for several alternative demonstration programs regarding insurance benefits for Medicare-eligible military retirees. In particular, section 722 authorized the DoD to implement a demonstration program known as the TRICARE Senior Supplement Demonstration. Under TSSD, certain Medicare-eligible DoD beneficiaries were offered the opportunity to enroll in TRICARE as a supplement to Medicare and to receive prescription drug coverage through the National Mail Order Pharmacy (NMOP) and TRICARE civilian network pharmacies. In Section 221 of the 1999 NDAA, Congress also authorized a parallel demonstration in which selected Medicare-eligible military retirees were eligible to enroll in the Federal Employees Health Benefit Program (FEHBP) as a supplement to Medicare. In addition, the NDAA of 2000 authorized the Uniformed Services Family Health Plan Continuous Open Enrollment Demonstration.[4] These demonstrations were designed to test possible models for providing supplemental insurance benefits to Medicare-eligible military retirees.

Eligible beneficiaries could enroll in TSSD beginning in spring 2000, and the demonstration was scheduled to end on December 31, 2002. TSSD is being conducted in and around Santa Clara County, California, and Cherokee County, Texas. An eligible beneficiary must reside in a defined area around these locations and must also be either a retiree of the Uniformed Services,

---

[2]This limitation followed the terms of Public Law 89-614, Military Medical Benefits Amendments of 1966, which established the Civilian Health and Medical Program of the Uniformed Services (CHAMPUS) and limited coverage to beneficiaries under 65.

[3] This is commonly referred to as "The Promise" by beneficiary organizations and even within TRICARE Management Activity (TMA), an office within the Department of Defense with responsibility for overseeing the administration of health benefits to military dependents and retirees.

[4]See Schoenbaum et al. (2001).

a dependent of a Uniformed Services retiree, or the dependent survivor of a Uniformed Services retiree or member.[5] Additionally, eligible beneficiaries are age 65 or over, are eligible for Medicare Part A, and are enrolled in Medicare Part B. Beneficiaries enrolled in TSSD are not eligible to receive care or pharmaceuticals from military health care facilities.

Congress directed the DoD to evaluate TSSD. Per the 1999 NDAA, the evaluation was to include the following:

1. An analysis of the costs of the demonstration project to the United States and to the eligible individuals who participate in such a demonstration project.

2. An assessment of the extent to which the demonstration project satisfies the requirements of such eligible individuals for the health care services available under the demonstration project.

3. An assessment of the effect, if any, of the demonstration project on military medical readiness.

4. A description of the rate of enrollment in the demonstration project of the individuals who were eligible to enroll in the demonstration.

5. An assessment of whether the demonstration project provides the most suitable model for a program to provide adequate health care services to the population of individuals consisting of the eligible individuals.

6. An evaluation of any other matters that the Secretary of Defense considers appropriate.

The DoD selected RAND to conduct this evaluation. This document represents RAND's final evaluation report.[6]

Overview of TRICARE for Life

During the course of TSSD, Congress passed the 2001 National Defense Authorization Act. Among other things, this law made sweeping changes to the way in which health care for Medicare-eligible military retirees is financed by directing the DoD to implement what is now commonly referred to as TRICARE

---

[5]The term *survivor* refers to either a dependent of a deceased Uniformed Services retiree or a dependent of a Uniformed Services member who died while serving on active duty for 30 days or more.

[6]In an unpublished project memorandum, RAND had previously reported to TMA regarding a subset of evaluation activities, particularly relating to focus groups conducted with TSSD enrollees and nonenrolled eligible beneficiaries (Cecchine et al., unpublished). The content of that preliminary memorandum is incorporated here, with appropriate notation, to make this final evaluation report as complete as possible.

for Life. As of October 1, 2001, TFL provides TRICARE as supplemental health insurance for all Medicare-eligible military retirees who are enrolled in Medicare Part B. In general, TFL covers all cost-sharing for Medicare-covered services and standard TRICARE cost-sharing for services that are covered by TRICARE but not by Medicare.

TFL provides Medicare-eligible military retirees with one of the most comprehensive health insurance benefits in the United States—with no monthly premium, no enrollment requirements, and coverage for some services not covered by Medicare (particularly prescription drugs)—and it is a permanent national program. TFL thus changed the policy context in which TSSD (and the FEHBP demonstration program) were taking place by preempting the possibility that the TRICARE Senior Supplement Demonstration program would be instituted in any permanent way.

Following the passage of the 2001 NDAA, RAND worked with the TRICARE Management Activity (TMA) to revise RAND's approach for evaluating TSSD. The goal was to identify ways in which the TSSD evaluation could inform policy toward eligible beneficiaries in the context of TFL. The revised evaluation plan is described in detail in Chapter 3, along with a description of elements of the original evaluation plan that were modified or deleted. The schedule for completing the evaluation was also accelerated, and the budget was reduced.

Organization of This Report

This chapter introduced the policy context within which TSSD was developed and implemented, including an overview of TRICARE for Life, a permanent national health insurance program available to all Medicare-eligible military beneficiaries as a supplement to Medicare as of October 2001. Chapter 2 provides more details about the health insurance options available to Medicare-eligible military beneficiaries prior to TSSD, through TSSD, and under TFL, and it describes the TSSD demonstration sites. Chapter 3 describes our evaluation methods. Chapters 4 and 5 present the results from focus groups that were convened and a beneficiary survey that was conducted as part of this evaluation. Chapter 6 provides a final discussion and conclusions regarding TSSD.

2. Background on Medicare, Supplemental Coverage, and TSSD

This chapter provides descriptions of the health insurance coverage options available to individuals eligible to participate in the TSSD program.

Health Insurance for Military Retirees (Prior to TFL)

The enactment of TFL substantially changed the health insurance options available to Medicare-eligible military retirees. The following sections describe options, including Medicare and Medicare supplements, available prior to TFL.

Medicare

Title XVIII of the Social Security Act, designated "Health Insurance for the Aged and Disabled," established a health insurance program for aged persons (commonly known as Medicare) to complement the retirement, survivors, and disability insurance benefits under Title II of the Social Security Act. Entitlement for Medicare is specified in 42 CFR 406. Most persons age 65 or over are eligible for Medicare.[1]

Medicare has traditionally consisted of two parts: Hospital Insurance (Part A) and Supplemental Medical Insurance (Part B). Part A coverage is generally provided automatically, free of premiums, to eligible persons. Beneficiaries must pay deductibles and copayments for inpatient hospital care and copayments for care in skilled nursing facilities. Coverage under Part B is based on voluntary enrollment and payment of a monthly premium ($54 for 2002). Eligible beneficiaries who do not enroll in Part B when they reach age 65 may do so at a later date. However, the Part B premium goes up 10 percent for each year after age 65 the beneficiary was not enrolled. For most outpatient medical services, Part B requires beneficiaries to pay 20 percent coinsurance, except for mental

---

[1]In addition, the following groups also became eligible for Medicare in 1973: persons entitled to Social Security or Railroad Retirement disability for at least 24 months (not applicable to the military retiree population), most persons with end-stage renal disease (ESRD), and certain otherwise non-covered aged persons who elect to pay a premium for coverage.

health services, which require 50 percent coinsurance. Medicare does not currently cover outpatient prescription drugs.

The Balanced Budget Act (BBA) of 1997 also introduced a third part, sometimes known as Part C, the Medicare+Choice program, which expanded beneficiaries' options for participation in private-sector health care plans.

Supplementing Medicare

To address the gaps in Medicare coverage, many Medicare beneficiaries, including Medicare-eligible military beneficiaries, have health insurance coverage that supplements Medicare. They obtain such coverage from a variety of sources, including private Medicare supplemental plans (commonly referred to as "Medigap" plans), plans sponsored by former employers, Medicare+Choice HMOs, Medicaid, and/or other public programs.

Private Medigap plans are standardized, with ten different benefit packages, referred to by the consecutive letters A through J.[2] All of these Medigap plans eliminate Medicare's coinsurance for inpatient care under Medicare Part A and outpatient care under Part B. In addition, they also reduce or eliminate out-of-pocket costs for other Medicare-covered services, with the types of services varying by plan; they also extend Medicare's benefit limits for certain services and/or cover some services that Medicare does not cover, with the types of benefits covered and the scope of coverage limited by the plan. Three of the plans (H through J) provide coverage for prescription drugs, up to a set dollar limit per year.

Employer-sponsored supplemental plans serve functions that are similar to those of private Medigap, although they generally include modest (although lower than Medicare's) cost-sharing requirements. At the same time, employer-sponsored plans generally include more-comprehensive coverage for prescription drugs than do private Medigap plans.

In addition, some Medicare beneficiaries enroll in HMOs under the Medicare+Choice program. Such plans reduce out-of-pocket expenses relative to fee-for-service Medicare; they also may offer additional benefits, such as transportation, eyeglasses, coordination of care, or prescription drugs. Premiums for Medicare+Choice plans tend to be substantially lower than the premiums for

---

[2] Summary information on the benefits in each of the ten standardized Medigap plans is available at http://www.medicare.gov/mgcompare/Search/StandardizedPlans/TenStandardPlans.asp.

Medigap plans. In recent years, many Medicare HMOs have withdrawn from the market. While most Medicare beneficiaries living in urban areas continue to have a Medicare HMO option, many beneficiaries in less urban or rural areas are not served by a Medicare HMO. Furthermore, even where Medicare HMOs remain available, the relative generosity of their benefits has decreased while the out-of-pocket costs for members have increased.

Private Medigap plans require beneficiaries to pay premiums, which vary by type of plan and, for most beneficiaries who enroll after age 65, by age and/or health status. Only three of the ten standardized Medigap policies include any prescription drug coverage; two of these currently have an annual benefit limit of $1,250, and the third has an annual limit of $3,000. We note that, historically, affinity organizations such as The Retired Officers Association and USAA, an association that provides insurance to military members and their families, offered basic Medigap plans to military retirees without medical underwriting. However, these offerings are limited to plans A through G, i.e., those without any prescription drug coverage. Employer-sponsored Medicare supplement plans may also require premiums, but this varies by employer. Medicaid and most other public programs require no premiums, but eligibility is based on beneficiaries' economic and/or health status. Medicare HMOs may also require premiums, which vary by plan.

Distribution of Health Insurance Coverage Among Military Retirees

We present the distribution of health insurance patterns for the TSSD population in subsequent sections. However, the two TSSD catchment areas may not be representative of the overall population of Medicare-eligible military beneficiaries, and we know of no definitive information on the nature and prevalence of Medicare supplemental coverage or Medicare+Choice enrollment in that population. For the general Medicare population, data suggest that relatively few Medicare beneficiaries have only Medicare (Table 2.1). For instance, the majority of Medicare beneficiaries whose income is above the poverty line have private supplemental insurance, via either a former employer or a Medigap policy. Roughly 11 percent have only Medicare. We note that Table 2.1 does not address the case of Medicare-eligible military retirees who live in the catchment areas of MTFs and receive care there; such care is provided at no charge to the beneficiary on a space-available basis.

Data from RAND's evaluation of the TRICARE Senior Prime Demonstration (another demonstration conducted in other locations, not to be confused with

Table 2.1

Health Insurance of Medicare Beneficiaries Aged 65+, 1997
(% of Medicare Beneficiaries)

	All Beneficiaries	<=100% of Poverty-Line Income	100%–200% of Poverty-Line Income	>200% of Poverty-Line Income
Employer/retiree	35	8	26	50
Medigap	25	15	28	27
Public	2	3	3	1
Medicare HMO	14	6	16	16
Medicaid	14	52	13	1
Medicare only	10	16	14	5

NOTE: Columns may not sum to 100% due to rounding. The Employer/retiree row includes both beneficiaries who have supplemental insurance from a former employer or union and those who are still working and whose employer is their primary source of insurance.

SOURCE: Urban Institute analyses of 1997 Medicare Current Beneficiary Survey, 2001.

TSSD) suggests that similar fractions of military retirees and other Medicare beneficiaries, respectively, were enrolled in Medicare+Choice plans in demonstration catchment areas prior to the demonstration.[3] It seems plausible that the fraction of military retirees who are covered by employer/retiree benefits may be lower than that for civilian Medicare beneficiaries due to different work histories (i.e., career employment with an employer—the DoD— that did not offer such coverage prior to TFL). RAND's TRICARE Senior Prime Demonstration evaluation also reported that approximately 7 percent of eligible beneficiaries in demonstration catchment areas were enrolled in Medicare Part A but not Part B because of the cost of Part B and beneficiaries' intentions to receive care from MTFs.

TSSD

As noted earlier, TSSD was designed to function as a Medigap policy. Table 2.2 summarizes some of the main features of TSSD, along with the corresponding Medicare features. Eligible beneficiaries could enroll in TSSD beginning on March 1, 2000, with coverage under the demonstration beginning on April 1, 2000. TSSD enrollees could disenroll at any time. The program was scheduled to end on December 31, 2002. However, all beneficiaries eligible for TSSD received pharmacy benefits under the new national pharmacy benefit program on April 1, 2001, and TFL benefits on October 1, 2001. Table 2.2 also summarizes the main features of TFL.

---

[3] See Farley et al. (2000). Under the Senior Prime Demonstration program, selected MTFs were qualified as Medicare+Choice HMOs, and Medicare-eligible military beneficiaries living in the catchment areas of these MTFs were eligible to enroll in these plans.

Table 2.2

Comparison of Plan Features for Medicare-Eligible Military Beneficiaries

Characteristic	Medicare (Fee-For-Service)[a]	TRICARE Senior Supplement	TRICARE For Life
Medicare supplemental coverage	No DoD-sponsored benefit	Yes	Yes
Main eligibility requirements	N/A	Age 65 or over and enrolled in Medicare Part B	Age 65 or over and enrolled in Medicare Part B
Enrollment required	Yes, for Part B	Yes	No
Premiums	None for Part A; $54/month for Part B[b]	$48/month (and Part B participation is required)	None (but Part B participation is required)
Outpatient cost-sharing	$100 annual deductible, plus 20% coinsurance for most outpatient care (50% for mental health care)	Covers most Medicare cost-sharing for covered services (coverage is generally higher for TRICARE network providers)	Covers all Medicare cost-sharing for TRICARE-covered services
Inpatient cost-sharing	Per-admission deductible for hospital care, plus copayments per day for stays longer than 60 days; also copayments for skilled nursing care for stays longer than 20 days	Covers most Medicare cost-sharing for covered services	Covers all Medicare cost-sharing for TRICARE-covered services
Coverage for TRICARE benefits not covered by Medicare	N/A	Yes, with TRICARE cost-sharing rules	Yes, with TRICARE cost-sharing rules
Pharmacy benefits	None under Medicare; no cost for prescriptions filled at MTF pharmacies; Base realignment and closure (BRAC) beneficiaries have access to NMOP	Yes, via NMOP and TRICARE network pharmacies (TSSD beneficiaries may not use BRAC drug benefits)	Yes, via new pharmacy benefit program; no cost for prescriptions filled at MTF pharmacies

10

Table 2.2—Continued

Characteristic	Medicare (Fee-For-Service)[a]	TRICARE Senior Supplement	TRICARE For Life
Provider network	No	Yes; lower cost-sharing when using TRICARE providers versus non-TRICARE Medicare provider	None for Medicare-covered services; lower cost-sharing when using TRICARE providers for other services covered by TRICARE
Automatic coordination of benefits with Medicare	N/A	Yes, for TRICARE network providers; No, for non-TRICARE providers (provider would bill patients for the balance due and patients would file claims with TSSD)	Yes
Catastrophic payment cap	No	Yes: $7,500 under TRICARE Standard	Yes: $3,000
Access to MTF clinical care[c]	On space-available basis, for beneficiaries in MTF catchment area; care provided at no cost to beneficiary	Not permitted for TSSD enrollees	On space-available basis, for beneficiaries in MTF catchment area; care provided at no cost to beneficiary

[a]Refers to coverage under fee-for-service Medicare in the absence of supplemental insurance benefits.

[b]For beneficiaries who did not enroll in Part B at age 65 but join later, their Part B premium is increased by 10% for each year after age 65 that they were not enrolled.

[c]Access to MTF primary care will be enhanced for participants in the DoD's new TRICARE Plus program. In addition, the temporary TRICARE Senior Prime Demonstration program provided comprehensive access to MTF care for participants.

Premiums and Cost-Sharing

TSSD benefits were more generous than any of the standard Medigap plans, particularly in regard to pharmacy benefits. TSSD premiums were $48 per month. In general, this premium amount was less than beneficiaries would have to pay for the most comparable private Medigap policy (Plan J), even if they enrolled at age 65 and were exempt from medical underwriting.

As a Medicare supplemental policy, TSSD covered most cost-sharing that beneficiaries would face under Medicare for Medicare-covered services.[4] The exact level of benefit depended on whether beneficiaries received care from TRICARE network providers (i.e., under TRICARE Extra) or from an authorized nonnetwork provider (i.e., under TRICARE Standard). For care from TRICARE network providers, TSSD would pay any cost-sharing remaining after Medicare (and any applicable Medigap policy) had processed the claim, up to the amount TRICARE would have paid if TRICARE had been primary payer. For care from nonnetwork providers, TSSD would pay an amount up to 115 percent of the TRICARE allowable charge, minus payments from Medicare and any applicable Medigap policy, up to the amount TRICARE would have paid if TRICARE had been the primary payer. TRICARE would bear no responsibility for billed charges in excess of 115 percent of the TRICARE allowable charge from nonnetwork providers. Beneficiaries would also need to meet applicable Medicare and TRICARE deductibles for outpatient care.

In addition, TSSD provided coverage for services that were covered by TRICARE but not Medicare, with TRICARE cost-sharing rules. TSSD also provided pharmacy benefits with modest cost-sharing rules and no annual benefit maximum (unlike private Medigap plans).

Other TSSD Characteristics

Several other characteristics of TSSD are worth highlighting because of their potential impact on enrollment:

- First, under TSSD (but not TFL), beneficiaries were required to forgo access to MTFs. However, the demonstration catchment areas were required to be located outside any MTF catchment area. In practice, most eligible beneficiaries were 100 or more miles from the nearest MTF, although a number of beneficiaries indicated that they drove long distances to use MTF pharmacies (see Appendix F).

- Second, also unlike TFL, Medicare did not coordinate claims with TSSD automatically as it does with most private and employer-sponsored Medigap plans. For patients receiving care from TRICARE network providers, the provider would file the claims. However, for patients receiving care from nonnetwork providers, in general providers would bill patients for the

---

[4]For TSSD enrollees who retained private or employer-sponsored Medigap coverage, TSSD would serve as third the payer, after the Medicare and the Medigap policy.

balance of the bill (after Medicare's payment) and patients would have to file claims with TSSD themselves.

- Finally, TSSD was a temporary program, and beneficiaries had no guarantee that it, or any analogous program, would be available at the end of the demonstration period (indeed, TFL was not enacted until well into the first year of TSSD, and it may not have begun to be widely understood by beneficiaries until the spring of 2001 with the dissemination of materials from the DoD and retiree organizations). Beneficiaries with private or employer-sponsored Medigap policies who enrolled in TSSD thus faced the decision of whether to continue their prior coverage and pay for both, or give up their prior coverage in favor of TSSD. In the latter case, beneficiaries risked the possibility that they would not be able to return to their prior plan or other comparable coverage at the end of the demonstration period, or that they would face medical underwriting if they did return.

The BBA of 1997 specifies conditions under which Medicare beneficiaries who enroll in a Medicare+Choice plan or a "similar organization operating under a demonstration project authority" are guaranteed access to certain Medigap plans. Text referring to these conditions was included in TSSD documents for beneficiaries, also available from the TRICARE Web site. However, it is likely that the provisions of the 1997 BBA do not apply to TSSD because it was not conducted under the demonstration authority of the Social Security Act (of which Medicare is a part) and because the relevant section (722) of the 1999 NDAA makes no mention of Medigap reinstatement.[5]

This issue is discussed in further detail in Chapter 4, particularly in the context of the focus groups we conducted with eligible beneficiaries.

Demonstration Sites

The 1999 NDAA specified that TSSD be conducted in two separate areas selected by the Secretary of Defense. Both areas were to be outside the catchment areas of any MTFs. One area was to have no Medicare+Choice plan coverage while the other was to have one or more of such plans available to Medicare beneficiaries. In practice, areas in and around Cherokee County, Texas, were selected as the area without Medicare managed-care penetration, while areas in and around Santa Clara County, California, were selected as the area with active

---

[5]This section is in specific contrast to section 721, which authorized the parallel FEHBP demonstration program in a section titled "Application of Medigap Protections to (FEHBP) Demonstration Project Enrollees."

Medicare+Choice plans. Cherokee County, southeast of Dallas, is relatively rural whereas Santa Clara County, close to San Jose, is relatively urban. Table 2.3 provides information on enrollment of Medicare beneficiaries in Medicare+ Choice HMOs in Santa Clara County in March 2000. See Appendix G for maps of the two TSSD demonstration areas.

As required, neither demonstration area is in the catchment area (i.e., within approximately 40 miles) of an MTF. The closest MTF to the Cherokee County area is at Barksdale Air Force Base in Louisiana, with an average travel distance of more than 90 miles (although some parts of the demonstration area are within 50 miles of Barksdale). The closest MTF to the Santa Clara County area is at Travis Air Force Base, with an average travel distance of more than 75 miles. We note that the Santa Clara demonstration area includes the Department of Veterans Affairs (VA) Palo Alto Medical Center. Parts of the Cherokee County area are within 25 miles of the VA's Lufkin Clinic; the closest VA Medical Center is in Shreveport, Louisiana.[6]

We did not formally assess the availability of TRICARE network providers in either demonstration area. However, we used the on-line TRICARE provider directory (www.tricare.osd.mil/ProviderDirectory/) to search for family practice physicians, cardiologists, and oncologists in randomly sampled zip codes in the

Table 2.3

Medicare+Choice HMO Enrollment, Santa Clara County

Plan Name	Number of Enrollees	Percentage of Medicare Eligibles	Percentage of Medicare+Choice Enrollees
Aetna US Healthcare of California	2,222	1.3	3.2
Blue Cross of California	1,665	1.0	2.4
California Physicians' Services Corporation	431	0.3	0.6
Health Net	6,167	3.6	8.8
Kaiser Foundation	37,832	22.1	54.0
Pacificare of California	23,917	14.0	34.1

SOURCE: Data on the general Medicare population for March 2000 is from the Health Care Financing Administration, http://www.hcfa.gov/medicare/mgd-rept.htm.

---

[6] We note that only a small subset of the population eligible for TSSD receive substantial amounts of care through the VA system. Spouses of veterans do not generally qualify for VA health care. Veterans are assigned a priority score based on the presence of service-connected disability, the nature of military service, and income. Roughly 37 percent of the nation's 26 million veterans have service-connected disabilities and/or sufficiently low incomes to receive free or very low-cost care through the VA (Department of Veterans Affairs, 1998). However, this fraction is lower among military retirees, due to their military pensions. Other veterans may use the VA but are required to pay substantial amounts for care comparable to Medicare copays and deductibles.

demonstration areas. In the Cherokee County area, it appeared that network providers were mainly available in the relatively large towns (e.g., Longview, Palestine, Nacogdoches) but not in more rural areas.[7] In the Santa Clara area, TRICARE network providers appeared to be relatively more prevalent, particularly in the San Jose/Palo Alto area where beneficiaries were most concentrated; provider density decreased substantially in the southern areas of the Santa Clara demonstration area, e.g., around Gilroy and Hollister.

---

[7]We note that these three towns are relatively far apart, e.g., 90 miles between Palestine and Longview, 78 miles between Palestine and Nacogdoches, and 71 miles between Longview and Nacogdoches.

3. Evaluation Methods and Data Sources

This chapter describes the methods we used to evaluate TSSD, along with evaluation components we had included in our original evaluation plan but dropped by agreement with the study's sponsor.

Overview of Evaluation Activities

At the beginning of the evaluation, RAND met with TMA project staff to develop and finalize an evaluation plan in order to meet the evaluation goals specified in the 1999 NDAA (and listed in Chapter 2). In practice, two factors required us to revise our initial evaluation plan. The first, discussed in greater detail later in this chapter, was the low rate of enrollment in the demonstration (total confirmed enrollment was 344 in September 2000 and 355 in November 2000, out of an eligible sample of approximately 11,000). The second factor was the passage of TFL, which substantially changed the context in which TSSD was being conducted. This section outlines our evaluation activities, along with activities that had been planned initially.

Briefings with Program Staff

RAND's evaluation began in May 2000. We began by meeting with TMA staff including Duaine Goodno, the TMA staff person responsible for overseeing the demonstration. TMA staff provided background materials on TSSD, including printed materials that had been distributed to eligible beneficiaries. Because RAND's evaluation began after the start of the demonstration, and particularly after the majority of TMA's efforts to publicize TSSD to eligible beneficiaries, we relied on TMA staff to describe the dissemination efforts.

TMA's publicity efforts were concentrated in the months preceding the initial enrollment period. The Iowa Foundation for Medical Care (the DoD contractor responsible for administering the demonstration) developed a database, drawn from the Defense Enrollment Eligibility Reporting System (DEERS), of all eligible beneficiaries in the demonstration areas. The Iowa Foundation mailed informational materials about TSSD to all eligible beneficiaries, and beneficiaries could obtain additional information by telephone. Mr. Goodno and representatives from the Iowa Foundation also visited the two demonstration areas and conducted "town meetings" at various locations to inform eligible beneficiaries about TSSD.

TMA informed us that they stopped marketing the demonstration to beneficiaries after the demonstration began because of administrative difficulties in administering the benefit and processing the claims (Goodno, 2000).

Automated Data Collection

TMA received monthly reports regarding TSSD enrollment and disenrollment from the Iowa Foundation for Medical Care. TMA forwarded these reports to us on a monthly basis. In addition, in preparation for direct data collection activities with beneficiaries, we requested and obtained data on all enrolled beneficiaries and on all eligible beneficiaries from the Iowa Foundation. These data are described in greater detail later in this chapter.

Our original evaluation design included a plan to obtain medical and pharmacy claims data on TSSD enrollees and on eligible beneficiaries from the Iowa Foundation, the DoD, and Medicare. However, the low enrollment in TSSD inhibited meaningful quantitative comparison between TSSD enrollees and nonenrolled eligibles (in particular due to the very skewed nature of health care expenditures, which makes a small sample very susceptible to outliers).[1] In addition, following the introduction of TFL, RAND and TMA agreed to restrict the scope of the evaluation and shorten its duration. Therefore, with the agreement of TMA, we eliminated the claims analysis.

Primary Data Collection

We conducted focus groups with TSSD enrollees and nonenrolled eligible beneficiaries to collect information about their attitudes toward the demonstration, their reasons for enrolling or remaining unenrolled, and information on other factors related to their enrollment. In addition, we conducted a mail survey of TSSD enrollees and nonenrolled eligible beneficiaries. Focus group and survey activities are described in greater detail in the remainder of this chapter.

We had originally anticipated sampling beneficiaries who had enrolled and then disenrolled from TSSD (for reasons other than death or relocation). However, the number of disenrollees was very small and did not support a separate analysis.

---

[1]See, for example, Sturm, Unutzer, and Katon (1999).

In the remainder of this chapter, we describe the design of the focus groups and the beneficiary survey.

Focus Group Design

There were two main goals for conducting focus groups as part of the TSSD evaluation: (1) to obtain qualitative information about the reasons why eligible beneficiaries enrolled or did not enroll in the demonstration program and to obtain opinions of and experiences with the demonstration in particular and the military health system in general and (2) to pilot test a survey questionnaire prior to administration to a larger sample of eligible beneficiaries.

Site Selection

Focus groups were conducted in each of the two demonstration areas: Santa Clara County, California, and Cherokee County, Texas. Selection of focus group sites in Santa Clara, California, and Longview, Texas, was based on the density of recently enrolled beneficiaries within a 15-mile radius, the availability of adequate facilities for conducting the focus groups, and the ease of access for participants.

Recruitment

Separate focus groups were used for TSSD enrollees and nonenrolled but eligible beneficiaries. The separate groups were used for two reasons: (1) because of the different relationships to the demonstration program of the two groups and (2) to avoid the discussion from turning into an informational meeting for nonenrollees.

For both sites, 30 enrollees and 30 nonenrollees were identified whose primary residence was within 15 miles of the focus group location. Data about beneficiaries were provided by the eligibility and enrollment files maintained by the Iowa Foundation for Medical Care. In several cases, more than 30 beneficiaries met these criteria, in which case 30 were selected randomly. For each focus group, sponsors[2] were twice as likely to be sampled as spouses were to ensure that no more than nine spouses would be included in any one focus group (to meet Office of Management and Budget [OMB] requirements).

---

[2] "Sponsors" in this context refers to persons whose military career qualifies them and their eligible dependents for health benefits.

Potential focus group participants received a recruitment letter from RAND accompanied by an endorsement letter from the study sponsor (see Appendixes A and B for sample letters). The endorsement letter was then followed by a phone call from RAND to confirm participation.

The goal was to confirm 12 participants for each focus group, with the expectation that 8 to 10 of them would actually attend. Recruitment and participation goals were met or surpassed for all focus groups (see Table 3.1).

Discussion Structure and Content

The focus group was divided into two parts: (1) the pilot test of the survey instrument and (2) a discussion guided by a set of interview questions developed in advance of the sessions (see Appendix C). Each focus group session began with introductions and a description of the purpose of the pilot test before the discussion commenced. Confidentiality issues were discussed and participants were reminded of the voluntary nature of their participation. RAND's Human Subjects Protection Committee approved the focus group protocol (see Appendix C).

Mail Survey Design

The main goal for conducting a beneficiary survey as part of the TSSD evaluation was to understand enrollment patterns by identifying characteristics that distinguished enrollees from nonenrollees. We were also interested in assessing beneficiaries' stated reasons for enrollment or disenrollment, beneficiaries' experiences with military-sponsored health care, and enrollees' experiences with TSSD.

In practice, our evaluation began after nearly all of the beneficiaries who would eventually enroll in TSSD had enrolled, and our survey was conducted after most enrollees had been participating in the program for more than six months. Because we were concerned about the accuracy of retrospective reporting of outcomes such as health care use, we were unable to collect data on health care use preceding the availability of, or enrollment in, TSSD.

Table 3.1

Focus Group Participants

		Number of Participants	
TSSD Site	Focus Group Date (2001)	Enrollee Focus Groups	Nonenrollee Focus Groups
Santa Clara County, California	January 23	16	8
Cherokee County, Texas	January 25	15	12

We initially proposed reinterviewing survey respondents in the second year of the demonstration to assess their experience with TSSD. However, this option was dropped due to the low enrollment in TSSD and due to the introduction of TFL.

Questionnaire Development

Development of the mail survey began in September 2000 with the identification of domains that would be examined in the survey. A draft instrument was developed using several sources for questions including the Medicare Current Beneficiary Survey and the Health Care Survey for Medicare-Eligible Military Retirees and Dependents. In particular, health status and service utilization items from these surveys were adapted to the TSSD questionnaire.

The survey was designed to elicit information on the respondent and his or her spouse's use of health care services, their stated preferences for health plan features, their current health insurance coverage, their knowledge of and experience with TRICARE, their attitudes toward military health care, and their health status (see Appendix E for a sample of the survey). Demographic information (e.g., income, education, and age) was also collected. The questionnaire was divided into seven sections as described in Table 3.2. In addition, the final page of the survey invited respondents to share any other comments they might have.

With the exception of the questions regarding health insurance coverage, the questionnaires for the two survey sites were identical. For California, the section of the questionnaire regarding the respondent's health insurance coverage asked specifically about Medicare HMO's, a health insurance option not available to the Texas study population.

Table 3.2

Topics Covered by TSSD Mail Survey

Section	Topic
A	Use of health care services by respondent
B	Opinion regarding health plan features and benefits
C	Current health insurance coverage of respondent
D	Respondent's knowledge of and participation in the TSSD program
E	Health status of respondent
F	Demographic information
G	Information regarding spouse's use of health care services, health plan coverage, participation in the TSSD program, and health status

Pilot Testing

To evaluate the questionnaire, a pilot version was administered to four focus groups that included 51 TSSD enrollees and eligibles. At the beginning of each focus group, participants were asked to complete the pilot questionnaire. They were instructed to flag any unclear or hard-to-answer questions with the page marker stickers that were supplied and to write any comments or questions on the margin next to the specific item. Participants were asked to spend up to 30 minutes on the pilot questionnaire. The participants were also told that they would have an opportunity to discuss with us at the end of the focus group session any questions or concerns they had regarding the questionnaire. The guided discussions that followed the pilot test focused on the factors that influenced participants' choice of health plans, their reasons for enrolling or not enrolling in TSSD, and their level of satisfaction with TSSD.

All participants in each of the four focus group sessions completed the survey. Participants completed the survey in 30 to 35 minutes, leaving roughly 40 minutes for discussion. Completion time did not appear related to enrollment status or demonstration site. Participants did not voice objections to the survey content or specific questions during or after the general discussion. None of the participants chose to stay after the end of the discussion to discuss the questionnaire in more detail.

Participants in each of the four groups marked questions requiring clarification. For example, some were confused as to whether MTF visits for medical treatment included pharmacy visits. Several areas in which participants had trouble following skip patterns were noted in reviewing completed pilot-tested questionnaires. The final version of the instrument was revised and simplified in light of these findings. The project team noticed that some of the respondents had difficulty turning the pages of the questionnaire. On the basis of this observation, the final version of the survey instrument was bound to ease page turning.

Other refinements to the instrument's language and skip patterns, as well as refinements to the order of sections and items within sections, were made prior to the main data collection.

Sampling

Our sample was drawn from two separate lists. The Iowa Foundation for Medical Care supplied the project team with data on individuals enrolled in the TSSD and on all beneficiaries eligible to enroll in TSSD. Core data elements came from DEERS, with enrollment status and updated contact information added by the Iowa Foundation. The files were current as of September 6, 2000, the date of the extracts.

Given the relatively small number of TSSD enrollees per site, all households with enrolled sponsors were sampled. Households with enrolled spouses but without enrolled sponsors were sampled subject to OMB regulations; these rules required us to contact no more than nine enrolled spouses directly without prior OMB approval of the data collection instrument and survey activities. Therefore, for the 15 spouses enrolled in TSSD and living in households with eligible but unenrolled sponsors, we surveyed the sponsor (the data collection instrument included a section on spouse's characteristics).[3] The enrollee sample included focus group participants because of the small total number of enrollees.

For the TSSD eligible group, only households with at least one eligible sponsor were sampled. To comply with OMB regulations, households with eligible spouses but no eligible sponsors were excluded from the study. Only one eligible sponsor per household was included in the sampling frame. Focus group participants and eligibles with enrolled spouses were excluded from the sampling frame.

Table 3.3 describes the sampling frame from which the study sample was selected. All 203 enrolled households (including 15 with enrolled spouses and nonenrolled sponsors) with adequate sponsor information—meaning that the

---

[3]A small number of TSSD enrollees consisted of spouses with no (eligible) sponsor in the household, either because the sponsor was not Medicare-eligible or because the sponsor was divorced or deceased. We did not survey these enrollees.

Table 3.3

Size and Composition of TSSD Sampling Frame and Sample

	Total Households	Excluded: No Sponsor Information	Spouse Only Enrolled[a]	Households in Sampling Frame[b]	Households Sampled
		Enrollees[c]			
California	75	18	7	57	57
Texas	174	28	8	146	146
Total	249	46	15	203	203
		Eligibles[d]			
California	5,866	1,840	N/A	4,026	825
Texas	2,379	584	N/A	1,795	825
Total	8,245	2,424	N/A	5,821	1,650

[a]Households in which the spouse has the same address as the sponsor.

[b]Equal to "total families" minus "families with no sponsor information" in the data files.

[c]Households in which *either* the sponsor or the spouse is enrolled in the TSSD program. Only the sponsor was eligible to receive the survey questionnaire. Only one sponsor per household was selected. Households that participated in the focus groups were *not* excluded.

[d]Households in which *neither* the sponsor nor the spouse is enrolled in the TSSD program. Only the sponsor was eligible to receive the survey questionnaire. Only one sponsor per household was selected. Households that participated in the focus groups were excluded.

data contained at least one name and a complete mailing address, and in the case of households with enrolled spouses, the spouse's address had to match the sponsor's address—were included in the sample. A random sample of 1,650 eligible households was selected from the 5,821 households in the sampling frame.

Data Collection

Data collection from the beneficiary survey began in March 2001 and was completed in June 2001. The study packet was sent to the sponsor of the selected household asking him/her to complete the questionnaire. The study packet included an advance letter, hard-copy questionnaire, and postage-paid return envelope. The packet also included an endorsement letter from the study sponsor. The enrollee sample was also divided into groups depending on whether the household had been invited to participate in the focus groups or not. A different advance letter was used for these two groups. (See Appendix A for samples of the recruitment letters.)

Table 3.4 lists the mailings to potential respondents, the dates of the mailings, and the response rates. Cases returned as undeliverable by the U.S. Postal Service (USPS) were not tracked any further. Respondents were deemed ineligible if they

Table 3.4

Response Rates by Fielding Task

Fielding Task	Sample Size	Dates (2001)	Response
First mailing	1,853	3/1–3/12	210 (11%)
Reminder letter	1,331	3/15–3/26	479 (36%)
Second mailing	981	3/27–4/5	454 (46%)
Third mailing	356	6/20–6/21	79 (38%)
Total	1,853[a]	3/1–6/21	1,222 (66%)

[a]As we describe later in this chapter, some beneficiaries were dropped from our sample frame due to death or relocation.

were deceased or moved out of the demonstration area (based on the list of Zip codes in the TSSD catchment area).

Phone prompts to nonrespondents (approximately 400 cases) were conducted from mid-May through mid-June. Nonrespondents received an average of two calls during this time period. Nonrespondents without phone numbers were tracked through directory assistance or a Web locator search engine. A number of survey packets were remailed as a result of the phone prompts. Completed surveys believed to have been returned in response to the third mailing pushed the overall response rate from 68 percent to 73 percent. Most of the converted nonresponses were from respondents in the TSSD eligible study group from both sites.

Table 3.5 provides a breakdown of survey participation. The response rate among TSSD enrollees was 95 percent (187 out of 197), whereas among TSSD eligibles it was 70 percent (1,035 out of 1,488). The undeliverable rate was

Table 3.5

Response Rates by Demonstration Site and Sample Type

Sample	N	Complete	Deceased	Out of Area[a]	Refusal	Other Non-response[b]	Response Rate[c]
California	882	552	57	31	32	210	70%
Enrolled	57	52	1	0	1	3	93%
Eligible	825	500	56	31	31	207	68%
Texas	971	670	47	33	39	182	75%
Enrolled	146	135	3	2	0	6	96%
Eligible	825	535	44	31	39	176	71%
Total	1,853	1,222	104	64	71	392	73%

[a]Cases no longer living in the program catchment area as determined by the zip codes of their new addresses provided by the USPS.

[b]Includes cases whose study packet was returned undelivered by the USPS because of a wrong address and for which no new address was provided; (n=140).

[c]Based on a study-eligible sample (excluding "Deceased" and "Out of Area"); (n=1,685).

8 percent of the sample eligible to respond to the survey. The out-of-area cases and deceased cases represented 3 percent and 6 percent of the entire sample, respectively. Overall, these cases (undeliverable, out of area, and deceased) were distributed fairly equally among the two sites but were more likely to occur among the TSSD eligible group than among the TSSD enrollee group because the contact information in the enrollee group was more likely to be current. Four percent of the sample who were eligible to respond to the survey actively refused to participate; about half of those cases were too old or too sick to complete the survey, while the remainder said they were not interested. Twelve cases returned separate written comments on various issues related to their health care coverage. An additional six completed surveys were received from TSSD-eligible respondents in California after the data collection period had ended.

We note that 58 percent (109 out of 187) of TSSD enrollees and 40 percent (405 out of 1,035) of TSSD eligibles provided some kind of write-in comments on the final page of their survey instrument. Anonymous survey comments on DoD health care policy are listed in Appendix F.

Data Quality

In this section, we discuss three issues related to the quality of the survey data.

Accuracy of Self-Reported Data. One issue related to the survey's data quality concerns the accuracy of self-reported TSSD enrollment. Of the 1,045 respondents we identified as not being enrolled in TSSD based on DEERS data, 33 reported on the survey that they were enrolled in TSSD (and, in general, answered the TSSD-specific questions in the survey). Similarly, of the 177 respondents we identified as enrolled in TSSD based on DEERS data, 9 reported on the survey that they were not enrolled in TSSD. These discrepancies may reflect a change in TSSD enrollment status between the time of the data extract and our field period and/or confusion between TSSD and TFL, which was generating substantial publicity especially in the second half of our field period. Finally, a small number of respondents identified themselves as uncertain as to whether they were enrolled in TSSD. In practice, however, the few who actually were enrolled, according to DEERS, completed the survey using the instructions for enrollees.

Table 3.6 provides more detail regarding DEERS versus self-reported data on TSSD enrollment. In practice, our analyses of survey data and health insurance

Table 3.6

Enrollment Patterns Among TSSD Survey Respondents (N=1,222)

Sponsor's Reports Regarding TSSD Enrollment Status	Total			Texas			California		
	Enrolled	Nonenrolled	Total	Enrolled	Nonenrolled	Total	Enrolled	Nonenrolled	Total
Sponsor enrolled	162	33	195	123	25	148	39	8	47
Sponsor not enrolled	9	985	994	4	494	498	5	491	496
Sponsor's enrollment uncertain	6	26	33	5	19	24	1	8	9
Spouse enrolled	107	33	140	82	27	109	25	6	31
Spouse not enrolled (or no spouse)	9	1,042	1,048	3	540	543	6	502	505
Spouse's enrollment uncertain	3	28	31	0	18	18	3	10	13

NOTE: Shaded cells indicate a conflict between sponsor reports and DEERS/Iowa Foundation data.

choice (described in Chapter 5) excluded beneficiaries whose TSSD enrollment status was inconsistent with DEERS data.[4]

Survey Nonresponse. A second issue related to the quality of the survey data is the rate of nonresponse. The overall rate of response of 73 percent seems acceptable, particularly for an elderly population. However, the response rate was significantly higher for households that included one or more TSSD enrollees than it was for those that did not. To examine these issues, we estimated a logistic regression using all sampled beneficiaries (excluding those we could identify as being deceased or having relocated out of the demonstration areas). The dependent variable was TSSD survey response. Explanatory variables included demographic variables available from the administrative data—i.e., age, race, gender, marital status, and state of residence—and TSSD enrollment status.

Table 3.7 provides predicted nonresponse rates associated with particular beneficiary characteristics based on the parameter estimates from this logistic regression. Each prediction is standardized for the values of all other covariates in the model.

Table 3.7 indicates that response rates rose significantly with age, that men were substantially more likely to complete the survey than women (although $p > 0.05$), and that unmarried respondents were significantly more likely to return the survey than those who were married. In addition, beneficiaries in Texas were significantly more likely to return the survey than those in California. Finally, the response rate was significantly higher for sponsors who were enrolled in TSSD relative to unenrolled sponsors with or without an enrolled spouse.

Differences in response rates, along with other unobservable differences between eligible beneficiaries who did or did not enroll in TSSD, respectively, will complicate any comparisons of insurance-related outcomes between enrollees and eligibles. Results of such quantitative analyses should therefore be interpreted cautiously.

Item Nonresponse. A third issue regarding the quality of the survey data is item nonresponse. Nonresponse varied by item but in general was low. For demographic characteristics and health characteristics, item nonresponse occurred with less than 5 percent of the respondents, and even for a relatively sensitive question such as one regarding household income, only 8 percent of respondents failed to give an answer.

---

[4]A small number of sponsors also reported that they were not eligible for Medicare, even though they were military retirees and age-eligible for Medicare. We also omitted these beneficiaries from most analyses.

Table 3.7

Predictors of Survey Nonresponse

Sponsor Characteristic	Fraction Not Responding	P-value of Contrast
Nonofficer	0.30	0.527
Officer	0.28	
White	0.29	0.481
Other	0.31	
Age 65–74	0.32	0.000
Age 75–84	0.28	
Age 85 and older	0.24	
Female	0.48	0.098
Male	0.29	
Unmarried	0.13	0.000
Married	0.32	
California	0.33	0.002
Texas	0.25	
Only sponsor enrolled	0.09	0.000
Only spouse enrolled	0.33	
Sponsor and spouse enrolled	0.13	
Neither enrolled	0.30	

NOTE: This table includes the predicted fraction of nonrespondents standardized for the covariates in the table. The sample includes all beneficiaries to whom we mailed a survey, excluding those who we subsequently learned were deceased or had moved out of the TSSD catchment area; (n=1,681).

Rather than delete a large number of cases with missing data, we imputed values for the missing items. For data elements, particularly demographics, that were available from DEERS, we imputed missing data using that information. To preserve sample size, particularly among TSSD enrollees, we imputed other key measures for survey respondents with item-nonresponse data by using the "impute" command in the Stata 7.0 statistical analysis package.[5]

---

[5] For each variable to be imputed, we specified a list of predictor variables, including a core set of demographic characteristics available on all beneficiaries from DEERS. Stata used these measures as explanatory variables in ordinary least squares regression models, with the measure to be imputed as the dependent variable. The imputed value was the prediction from the regression model for beneficiaries with a missing value of the dependent variable and nonmissing values of the predictors.

4. Focus Group Findings

The focus groups of TSSD enrollees and eligible nonenrollees were previously described in a project memorandum for TMA (Cecchine et al., unpublished). We repeat the main substantive findings of that memorandum in this chapter. Conclusions from the focus group findings are incorporated into Chapter 6.

Results for Nonenrollees

This section presents results from the nonenrollee focus group, including findings on nonenrollees' current coverage, factors related to their choice of plan, and their reasons for nonenrollment.

Current Health Insurance Coverage

All of the participants in the Texas group were enrolled in Medicare plus another insurance plan. The majority of them mentioned having private Medigap policies. Several specifically mentioned having purchased supplemental policies through advocacy or service organizations. Several were in an employer-sponsored plan offered by a former or current employer. One participant mentioned having Medicare and Medicaid. None of the Texas participants mentioned being enrolled in an HMO, reflecting a lack of Medicare risk contracts in the region. However, some participants reported that their employer supplements restricted their choice of doctor and hospital.

By contrast, roughly one-half of the California participants were enrolled in a Medicare HMO (Secure Horizons or Kaiser), reflecting the regional presence of Medicare HMOs. The remaining California attendees were enrolled in Medigap insurance, either through an advocacy or service organization or via an employer-sponsored plan.

Factors Influencing Choice of Plan

At both sites, coverage and cost were the most frequently mentioned factors influencing participants' choice of health plans, mostly in relation to prescription drugs. Being able to choose one's own physician and hospital were also commonly mentioned in both sites. California participants expressed dissatisfaction with their current HMO and the desire for greater access to MTF providers. Participants mentioned turning to Medicare HMOs for prescription drug coverage after the MTF at Moffett Air Force Base (AFB) closed because other MTFs were either too far away or required long waits for pharmacy service. California participants specifically mentioned long waits for pharmacy service at Travis AFB because of the large number of retirees already living in the catchment area. Individuals at both sites expressed difficulty in getting prescriptions filled at MTFs, which stemmed, in part, from the amount of paperwork involved.

It was unexpected that participants in Texas would indicate that factors related to provider choice influenced their choice of health plan because of the lack of managed care organizations in rural Texas. Although the focus group leaders did not probe participants further on this issue, the participants' responses indicated a high degree of sensitivity to issues of provider access. Participants in California seemed most sensitive to cost and prescription drug issues and voiced a general distrust of HMOs. The following selected responses from both locations reflect factors influencing plan choice:

> Being able to choose my own physician is most important.

> I like to know which hospital and physician I can use.

> Spousal coverage is important.

> HMOs are a scandal. This is wrong. This is evil that you would make a profit off somebody's suffering. They're not there to help anybody; they're there to make money.

Awareness and Knowledge of TSSD

Only four of the Texas participants said they had heard about the demonstration prior to attending the focus group. Those who were aware of the program had either attended the informational meeting at Barksdale AFB or a town hall meeting at the local Veterans of Foreign Wars chapter. Others mentioned reading about the program in military-related publications but lacked any understanding of its details. The majority of California participants had heard of TSSD through a service-related organization, but several had no knowledge of it at all.

Reasons for Not Enrolling in TSSD

Discussions at both sites suggested that the temporary nature of the demonstration and expected difficulties in reinstating Medigap coverage served as strong deterrents to enrollment. Participant comments, particularly those in Texas, suggested a fundamental lack of understanding of the program.

Several Texas participants were reluctant to risk losing the insurance coverage that they currently had after the demonstration ended. Similarly, California participants mentioned the fear of being unable to return to prior Medigap coverage because of preexisting-condition clauses. One Texas participant mentioned that the program did not really offer access to all of the health benefits available to other military personnel through the military health system. Another participant currently covered by an employer-sponsored plan indicated that it was difficult to understand how this program worked for spouses. Participants in both sites were unsure how the military benefits would work with the other insurance that they might have.

Several Texas participants indicated that they would *not* join the program, even if TSSD were permanent, for a number of reasons—covered benefits were not clearly defined, the distances they needed to travel to receive care were too long, and the pool of doctors available to program participants was too limited. These comments may indicate that some of the nonenrollees confused the TSSD program with TRICARE Prime or perhaps the TRICARE Senior Prime Program (another demonstration conducted in other locations). The following selected responses are from both locations:

> There were 500 people at the meeting over at Barksdale and 495 walked out. It was unreal. Once you switch over you cannot go back [to your Medigap].

> Most of us chose not to do it because we'd like to keep what we have.

> They can't guarantee [coverage] past two years. The program wasn't widely used because people were afraid of what would happen after then.

> I went to the seminar. I didn't join because I didn't trust them. I'm not going to cancel out my doctor [only to] have them fold.

> If I cancel my supplement I can't go back.

> I'm happy with my current insurance [even if it is more expensive].

> I [an informational meeting attendee] couldn't find anyone who would tell me what my wife's status would be if I switched over to TRICARE.

> I would have joined if it were permanent like the new one [TRICARE for Life].

> I would have signed up if I had received information about it. The benefits were not defined, and I was not about to drop my supplemental to try something [that] some politician could later decide was too costly.

I would not have joined because there are no TRICARE doctors where I
live.

Good doctors won't accept TRICARE.

TRICARE does not pay its doctors in a timely manner.

The problem is that TRICARE is a government program.

[TSSD] was never offered to me.

Dissatisfaction with Military Health Benefits

Nonenrollees' lack of familiarity with TSSD and their general dissatisfaction with
their health insurance coverage made it difficult to focus the discussion as the
protocol intended. Instead, nonenrollees preferred to talk about their distrust of
the government and unhappiness with military health care benefits. Common
themes focused on a "broken promise" by the DoD to provide lifetime health
care to retirees and their feelings of having been abandoned by the government.
The following selected responses are from both locations:

> TRICARE is going to have to come out with something that beats the
> dickens out of Medicare and a supplement in order for us to fall in line
> with [it] and to abandon what we've got and crawl in bed with TRICARE.

> They closed too many MTFs.

> We are not talking about health care; we are talking about money.

> We don't need a program; we need an address where we can send bills to
> and they pay them.

> What we [are] looking forward to is like the medical center in San Antonio.
> A guy gets sick down there, he goes to the hospital, and gets everything
> taken care of. He doesn't pay a penny out of his pocket. Why can't we do
> that out here?

> I can't get the medications I need at Barksdale. They tell me I have to see a
> civilian doctor.

> They waited for most of us to die off and now they've come out with this.

Impact of a Stand-Alone Drug Benefit on Interest in TSSD

To qualitatively determine the importance of drug coverage as a factor
influencing interest in TSSD, participants were asked to speculate on how the
availability of a stand-alone low-cost prescription drug benefit offered by the
military health care system would affect their interest in TSSD. It is possible that

some nonenrollees might prefer to remain enrolled in their current Medigap plan if the DoD provided a stand-alone drug benefit such as that available to BRAC beneficiaries. However, this question was quite difficult for the participants to answer for several reasons. First, questions involving hypothetical options are difficult to answer in general. Second, nonenrolled participants were not familiar enough with TSSD to make an informed judgment. Third, it was difficult for participants to draw the distinction between the TSSD program and the new, expanded drug coverage provided under the 2001 National Defense Authorization Act.

Notwithstanding these potential sources of confusion, many participants indicated that they would be interested in getting their prescriptions through such a benefit and might prefer that method to joining a TRICARE Medigap plan. The following selected responses are from both locations:

> It takes a long time and it's a hassle to get the medications I need.

> A drug benefit does not help me because I get that through my employer.

> Drug benefits are the main thing I am interested in.

> My wife's prescription drug benefit is $12 more a month than my retired pay.

Impact of Space-Available Care on Interest in TSSD

To qualitatively assess the importance of MTF care on participants' preferences, participants were asked to speculate on the effect expanded space-available care at the closest MTF would have on their interest in TSSD. Although this question was hypothetical, it proved easier to answer than the question on how a drug benefit might influence their interest in TSSD. Overall, the idea of receiving care at MTFs was attractive to participants in both sites. However, Texas participants, who must travel roughly 65 miles to the nearest MTF, indicated that travel distance would remain an important practical barrier even if access to space-available care were expanded.

Participants in California, where travel distances to MTFs are shorter, expressed a desire to receive more MTF care because they perceive that care to be of high quality and feel that MTF providers are more likely to have their patients' best interests at heart than are civilian HMO providers. However, some participants in California pointed out that traveling to an MTF becomes more difficult with age. As a result, space-available care would benefit mostly those who are just entering retirement and are better able to travel. The following selected responses are from both locations:

It's too far to travel, [and after you get there] you sit around all day.

When you are sick you don't feel like traveling to see a doctor.

Military doctors are good doctors.

Senior Prime is limited. Why can't it be available [all] over the country?

Other Issues

Overall, the sentiment of the group was that Congress cannot be trusted to keep TRICARE as an option for military retirees, despite the promise of health care for life they believe the government made to them when they entered a uniformed service.

Participants in California suggested that in their experience many doctors do not accept TRICARE because of problems with getting reimbursed in a timely manner. They also suggested that doctors who do accept TRICARE patients are not considered to be of high quality.

Many participants reiterated that a good prescription drug benefit available through the military would be highly valued. However, some voiced concern about the completeness of the formulary for geriatric care.

Finally, a participant in California indicated that having health coverage through the military after his/her sponsor dies is a "life saver."

Results for TSSD Enrollees

This section presents the results from focus groups conducted with TSSD enrollees, including findings on the factors affecting their choice of health plans, their experiences with TSSD thus far, and their perceptions of interest in the program among eligible beneficiaries.

Factors Affecting Choice of Plan

Participants mentioned low monthly premiums, the ability to choose one's own physician, and low out-of-pocket costs for prescription drugs as important factors influencing their choice of a health plan. Several also mentioned their desire to have military-sponsored health care. A minority did not identify any particular factor but instead indicated that their decisionmaking process was less structured than that of other participants. One participant said:

> I signed up in this program without having the foggiest notion what I'm doing in it. I never had anybody explain what [TSSD] amounts to.

Experience Thus Far with TSSD

Enrollees in both sites reported a high degree of satisfaction with the demonstration to date. One participant said his dependent spouse was "delirious" (happy) with TSSD. Enrollees expressed the greatest satisfaction with the drug benefit and the low premiums as compared with commercial Medigap plans.

Although administrative hassles seemed to be lessening over time, they were the biggest sources of dissatisfaction at both sites. Participants at both sites suggested that there needs to be better coordination between TSSD and Medicare. They noted that TSSD did not appear to be connected electronically to Medicare, as is the case with other Medigap carriers. A California participant pointed out that there is an option to file claims electronically and this option works well, although few providers accept it.

Participants in Texas indicated that it is not easy to find a provider that accepts TSSD. Some suggested that TRICARE administrators are not aware of TSSD and have therefore processed claims incorrectly. For example, one participant related a story of how TRICARE initially refused to cover the cost of a prescription. A TRICARE representative told him that he was no longer covered by TRICARE because he was over age 65. A California participant stated that he has claims that have been unresolved for months. Another participant speculated that claims are often processed incorrectly because TSSD is confused with other TRICARE programs. Similarly, Texas participants suggested that providers and TRICARE administrators confuse TSSD with TRICARE Prime.

Several participants reported problems in getting their prescriptions filled because of delays in entering enrollees into the DoD's computer system. However, getting reimbursed for the cost of those prescriptions was not mentioned as being a problem.

The following selected responses related to TSSD administration are from both locations:

> People at TRICARE Southwest want to treat TSSD like TRICARE Prime and that's not the program. TSSD needs a computer link to Medicare to pay claims directly.

> Every other supplement is linked electronically to Medicare, but not TRICARE.

You will get letters telling you that you owe the copayment.

The office that pays the bills is misinforming hospitals. They tell hospitals that the individual is over 65 and not allowed to participate in TRICARE. I've had to tell them to straighten out these individuals.

They looked at the temporary plastic card like it was counterfeit.

It would help this program if they gave information to caregivers that this is TSSD and not TRICARE Prime.

Providers look at the program as TRICARE, rather than as a Medicare supplement. They don't understand the difference between TRICARE and CHAMPUS.

Everything in the booklet I have says TRICARE Prime.

I file my own claims because my doctor won't take TRICARE. I sent a claim in October 19th. I got a reply December 10th. That's the average reply time.

They ask for the same things over and over [e.g., a copy of a Social Security card].

I made ten phone calls and wrote letters [to resolve a claim], but you still just go around in circles.

They [TRICARE administrators] seem to not realize that [TSSD] is a supplement program and not a freestanding insurance plan.

The following selected responses related to the TSSD pharmacy benefit are from both locations:

The pharmacy benefit is great.

A pharmacy in town told me I was not covered by TRICARE because I am over 65. When I got home I called TRICARE, [and] they told me that I had to get into the system. When I returned the next day, I was in the system.

Once you are in the system, everything is okay.

I have trouble finding TRICARE qualified providers.

The Mail Order Program has been a miracle to me.

The Mail Order Program is the best thing going.

You can't beat the $8 copay.

Even the 20% you pay at the drugstore is a great deal.

They don't cover everything [e.g., estrogen patches are covered, but estrogen injections are not].

Perceptions of Interest in TSSD Among Program Eligibles

We asked enrollees why more people have not enrolled in the TSSD program. Participants in both sites cited similar factors, such as the following:

- Many eligible beneficiaries said they have better coverage through their employer or can afford plans with better coverage or a better benefits package.

- Many eligible beneficiaries said they were not knowledgeable about the program. Participants at both sites reported that the informational meeting was not well publicized and not everyone received a letter advertising the meeting.

- Participants in Texas suggested that many eligible beneficiaries probably did not want to drop their current Medigap coverage.

- Many physicians who do not accept TRICARE confused TSSD with TRICARE and told patients that they did not accept that form of insurance. (One attendee in Texas claimed that all of the literature he had received regarding TSSD had the TRICARE Prime title and logo on it.)

- Participants reported that TRICARE does not have a good reputation for paying doctors promptly.

- Many eligible beneficiaries said they do not trust the government and are upset that they are not getting the free care they were promised.

Impact of a Stand-Alone Drug Benefit on Interest in TSSD

As with the nonenrollees, participants had a difficult time answering the question on how a drug benefit might influence their interest in TSSD. The participants equated a "stand-alone" drug benefit with an expanded benefit administered through MTFs. Nonetheless, the answers provide insight into the perceived incremental value of TSSD over alternative approaches for expanding DOD health benefits to Medicare-eligible retirees.

In general, the notion of a stand-alone drug benefit was attractive to most of the participants. However, many participants, particularly in California, indicated that TSSD is better than a stand-alone benefit because it provides more than just pharmacy coverage at a low cost, which would necessitate some type of Medigap insurance for catastrophic coverage. The following responses from enrollees address the stand-alone drug benefit:

> I would prefer [TSSD]. I would still need a supplement and this supplement is half the cost of the one I had.

> Keep what we have and make it better.

Impact of Space-Available Care on Interest in TSSD

Overall, the enrolled participants expressed somewhat less interest than nonenrollees in using MTF providers in lieu of TSSD. As with the nonenrollees, enrolled participants in Texas preferred TSSD to expanded space-available care because the closest MTF was too far away. The availability of no-cost prescription drugs was perceived as the major benefit of receiving care at MTFs; however, Texas participants added that the limited MTF formulary made MTF care less attractive. Others noted that the advantage of no-cost prescriptions at MTFs was offset by the option to use the mail order pharmacy program (the NMOP) as part of TSSD.

The following selected responses are from both locations:

> There are not that many bases close to us.

> I would prefer this program. I'm not allowed to travel that far.

> People in San Antonio are not happy with care in military facilities.

> This program is better because I have the freedom to go to any doctor I choose to.

> The Barksdale [MTF] is only a small clinic and not a hospital. They don't have all the staff and drugs we need.

Temporary Nature of the Demonstration

Given the level of apprehension expressed by nonenrollees about the risk associated with dropping current Medigap policies to enroll in a temporary demonstration program, enrollees in Texas were asked how the temporary nature of the demonstration affected their interest in the program. Compared with nonenrollees, TSSD enrollees in Texas expressed a high degree of confidence that (1) the program would be made permanent or (2) they would be able to reinstate their Medigap coverage in the event that the program was not made permanent.

The confidence the participants expressed about their ability to return to their Medigap plans at the termination of the demonstration was somewhat surprising, given the imprecise language on the topic on page four of the

TRICARE Senior Supplement Demonstration handbook (Department of Defense/TRICARE Management Activity, n.d.). The participants attributed their confidence to reassurances given to them in informational meetings conducted by TMA staff and contractors in which DOD representatives "promised" participants that their insurance companies would "take them back" at the end of the demonstration. This confidence may also be traced to the large proportion of this population having Medigap plans with no prescription drug benefits and that are sold by retiree organizations such as The Reserve Officers Association (TROA) without medical underwriting.

The following selected responses are from participants in Texas:

> Before I dropped our other supplement, I made sure that I could get back into our old supplement. I made them give me a letter.

> A lot of people walked out of the meeting at Barksdale once they found out that the program was temporary.

> When I found out the program was temporary, I did not enroll right away.

> At that meeting, they promised that the insurance company would have to take you back.

> I remember what the guy from the Pentagon told us. He said these programs have a way of going only [one of] three ways. They get expanded, they get extended, or made permanent. And besides, I understand you've got an open enrollment period with Medigap if it folds up.

> TROA promised to take us all back if [the TSSD] folds.

5. Mail Survey Findings

In the first part of this chapter, we present descriptive cross-tabulations of beneficiary characteristics by TSSD enrollment status and state of residence. Because there may be a possible correlation among characteristics that affect TSSD enrollment, we also examine TSSD enrollment and health insurance choice using multivariate models that control for various characteristics simultaneously. We did this to identify those characteristics that are independently associated with health plan choice. Our multivariate models include tests of statistical significance.

All data are based on sponsor reports in the beneficiary survey, except for the data regarding TSSD enrollment status, which are also assessed using DEERS/Iowa Foundation data (see Chapter 3). For tabulations and models that combine enrollees and nonenrollees, we weighted respondents by the inverse of the probability that they were sampled (in practice, the relative weights are 1.0 for enrollees and 3.5 for nonenrollees).

Enrollment Patterns

Table 5.1 reports TSSD enrollment patterns among survey respondents based on DEERS/Iowa Foundation data. As noted in Chapter 3, for a small number of sponsor and spouse respondents, their DEERS and self-reported TSSD enrollment status did not correspond. Those respondents are included in Table 5.1 but are excluded from the remaining analyses in this chapter.

The overall TSSD enrollment rate among our survey respondents was 3.6 percent of eligible sponsors. The enrollment rate was more than twice as high in the Texas demonstration area as in the California area. (As we will discuss further in this chapter, with respect to our multivariate models, California beneficiaries were more likely to be enrolled in private or employer-sponsored Medigap plans—including Medicare HMOs—than were beneficiaries in Texas).

Approximately two-thirds of responding sponsors were married to a spouse who was also eligible for TSSD (marital status independent of spousal eligibility is reported separately later in this chapter). In households with two eligible beneficiaries, typically either both or neither spouse was enrolled in TSSD.

Table 5.1

Enrollment Patterns Among Survey Respondents, Based on DEERS Status

	Total		Texas		California	
	Unweighted Number	Fraction of Subtotal	Unweighted Number	Fraction of Subtotal	Number	Fraction of Subtotal
All sponsors	1,222	—	670	—	552	—
Sponsor enrolled in TSSD	177	0.036	132	0.052	45	0.019
Sponsor not enrolled in TSSD	1,045	0.964	538	0.948	507	0.981
Sponsors without eligible spouse	423	—	229	—	194	—
Sponsor enrolled in TSSD	48	0.035	33	0.046	15	0.023
Sponsor not enrolled in TSSD	375	0.965	196	0.954	179	0.977
Sponsors with eligible spouse	799	—	441	—	358	—
Sponsor and spouse enrolled in TSSD	106	0.043	82	0.064	24	0.021
Only sponsor enrolled in TSSD	23	0.009	17	0.013	6	0.005
Only spouse enrolled in TSSD	10	0.004	3	0.002	7	0.006
Neither sponsor nor spouse enrolled in TSSD	660	0.943	339	0.921	321	0.968

NOTE: This table and the following tables in this chapter present the actual number of survey respondents in each category. However, fractions are weighted to reflect sampling probabilities and specifically our oversampling of households with TSSD enrollees.

Sample Characteristics

Table 5.2 reports data on the demographic characteristics of survey respondents by TSSD enrollment status and state of residence. We note that the sample size of enrollees—sponsors and spouses—is relatively small, particularly in California. For this reason, and because enrollees and nonenrollees presumably differ in unobservable ways as well, patterns between enrollees and nonenrollees should be interpreted cautiously.

Enrolled sponsors are more likely to be married than those who are not enrolled (and, as noted earlier, their spouses are substantially more likely to be enrolled in TSSD as well). Relative to the nonenrolled sponsors, enrolled sponsors were somewhat more likely to be white, less likely to be black, and less likely to have had some college.

Table 5.2

Demographic Characteristics of TSSD Survey Sample, Sponsors

	All Sponsors[a]			Enrolled Sponsors			Nonenrolled Sponsors		
	All	TX	CA	All	TX	CA	All	TX	CA
N (sample size)	1,180	641	539	168	128	40	1,012	513	499
Male	0.98	0.99	0.98	0.98	0.98	0.98	0.98	0.99	0.98
Mean age in years	74.1	72.9	75.3	73.4	73.1	74.6	74.1	72.9	75.3
Standard deviation	*6.0*	*5.6*	*6.2*	*5.6*	*5.3*	*6.3*	*6.0*	*5.6*	*6.2*
Mean number of people in household	2.1	2.0	2.2	2.1	2.1	2.2	2.1	2.0	2.2
Standard deviation	*1.2*	*0.8*	*1.6*	*0.8*	*0.7*	*1.0*	*1.2*	*0.8*	*1.6*
Married	0.80	0.82	0.79	0.88	0.88	0.88	0.80	0.82	0.79
Spouse enrolled in TSSD[b]	0.06	0.07	0.04	0.83	0.84	0.78	0.02	0.01	0.02
Race/Ethnicity									
Non-Hispanic white	0.78	0.87	0.70	0.85	0.87	0.78	0.78	0.87	0.70
Non-Hispanic black	0.05	0.03	0.07	0.01	0.01	0.00	0.05	0.03	0.07
Hispanic	0.03	0.00	0.05	0.02	0.00	0.08	0.03	0.00	0.05
Other	0.05	0.01	0.10	0.02	0.02	0.05	0.05	0.01	0.10
High school or less	0.70	0.81	0.58	0.60	0.65	0.44	0.70	0.82	0.58
Mean household income (in $1,000s)	50.1	41.5	59.5	49.9	44.5	68.3	50.1	41.3	59.3
Standard deviation	*27.2*	*22.6*	*28.7*	*25.5*	*22.4*	*27.0*	*27.3*	*22.6*	*28.7*
Officer at time of retirement	0.38	0.28	0.48	0.58	0.54	0.73	0.37	0.26	0.47
Belongs to military retiree organization	0.52	0.51	0.53	0.65	0.67	0.56	0.51	0.50	0.53
Medicare-eligible (self-reported)	0.95	0.96	0.93	0.99	0.99	0.98	0.95	0.96	0.93

NOTE: In this table and the tables that follow, the numbers indicate fractions of the sample, unless otherwise noted (e.g., sample size, standard deviation).

[a] Weighted to reflect differential probability of sampling for enrollees and nonenrollees.

[b] "Not enrolled" includes households with no spouse or with a spouse who is not age-eligible for TSSD.

In both Texas and California, mean household income is higher among enrollees than it is among nonenrollees; however, the difference between all enrollees and nonenrollees is relatively smaller than it is between enrollees in each state, apparently as an artifact of income differences between Texas and California and the relatively low rate of TSSD enrollment in California. Similar differences are evident with regard to officer status at the time of retirement, with enrollees being significantly more likely to have retired as an officer (or warrant officer) than are nonenrollees. Finally, enrollees are more likely to be members of military retiree organizations.

Health Insurance, Health Care Usage, and Health Status

Table 5.3 presents information on health insurance, health care usage, and health status by TSSD enrollment status and state of residence. Among nonenrollees, about 30 percent had only Medicare coverage as their source of health insurance,[1] nearly one-half had privately purchased Medigap coverage (and/or, in California, coverage through a Medicare+Choice HMO), and approximately one-quarter had employer-sponsored supplemental coverage. Compared with the national data on the general Medicare population, which was reported in Table 2.1, our survey respondents had lower rates of employer-sponsored supplemental coverage and public insurance, similar rates of private Medigap/HMO coverage, and higher rates of Medicare coverage without any supplement. About one-half of nonenrollees reported having some kind of prescription drug benefit, but the fraction was twice as high in California than it was in Texas, presumably due to Medicare HMOs.

For TSSD enrollees, the survey assessed their health insurance coverage prior to TSSD enrollment. Nearly two-thirds of Texas enrollees, and one-third of California enrollees, had previously held private Medigap policies. Approximately 18 percent of California enrollees had been in an HMO, including HMOs in Medicare+Choice plans and employer coverage provided via an HMO; a similar fraction of California enrollees, but only 6 percent of Texas enrollees, reported having previously had employer-sponsored coverage. Finally, half of the California enrollees, but only 13 percent of the Texas enrollees, reported having had pharmacy benefits previously.

---

[1]The TSSD survey asked beneficiaries about Medicaid, but it neglected to assess eligibility for VA benefits. Some beneficiaries specified VA coverage under "other" insurance. In practice, the total number of beneficiaries with Medicaid, VA, or other government-sponsored benefits was too small to examine separately.

Table 5.3

Sponsors' Health Insurance, Health Care Usage, and Health Status

	All Sponsors[a]			Enrolled Sponsors			Nonenrolled Sponsors		
	All	TX	CA	All	TX	CA	All	TX	CA
N (sample size)	1,180	641	539	168	128	40	1,012	513	499
Current health insurance									
Medicare or Medicare+Public	—	—	—	—	—	—	0.29	0.34	0.24
Private supplemental or HMO	—	—	—	—	—	—	0.45	0.43	0.47
Employer sponsored	—	—	—	—	—	—	0.26	0.23	0.29
TSSD	—	—	—	1.00	1.00	1.00	—	—	—
Currently have prescription drug coverage	—	—	—	1.00	1.00	1.00	0.54	0.39	0.74
Insurance prior to TSSD									
Private Medigap	—	—	—	0.60	0.70	0.32	—	—	—
Medicare HMO	—	—	—	0.05	0.00	0.18	—	—	—
Employer	—	—	—	0.10	0.06	0.21	—	—	—
Medicaid	—	—	—	0.00	0.00	0.00	—	—	—
Other	—	—	—	0.23	0.21	0.32	—	—	—
None	—	—	—	0.11	0.09	0.18	—	—	—
Previously had prescription drug coverage	—	—	—	0.213	0.133	0.484	—	—	—
Any hospital stay in past year	0.22	0.22	0.22	0.25	0.24	0.26	0.22	0.22	0.22
Any emergency room visit in past year	0.31	0.31	0.31	0.27	0.24	0.39	0.31	0.31	0.31
Mean number of physician visits in past year	5.9	6.0	5.7	5.8	5.7	6.0	5.9	6.0	5.7
Standard deviation	*4.1*	*4.1*	*4.1*	*3.9*	*3.9*	*3.8*	*4.1*	*4.1*	*4.1*
Currently use prescription drugs (mean number of prescription medications)	4.1	4.4	3.8	3.8	3.8	3.9	4.1	4.4	3.8
Standard deviation	*2.2*	*2.2*	*2.1*	*2.2*	*2.1*	*2.3*	*2.2*	*2.2*	*2.1*

46

Table 5.3—Continued

	All Sponsors[a]			Enrolled Sponsors			Nonenrolled Sponsors		
	All	TX	CA	All	TX	CA	All	TX	CA
General health status									
Excellent	0.12	0.11	0.13	0.20	0.19	0.26	0.12	0.10	0.13
Very good	0.28	0.25	0.32	0.30	0.31	0.28	0.28	0.25	0.32
Good	0.32	0.32	0.33	0.28	0.28	0.31	0.32	0.32	0.33
Fair	0.18	0.22	0.14	0.14	0.15	0.10	0.18	0.22	0.14
Poor	0.09	0.10	0.07	0.06	0.07	0.05	0.09	0.10	0.07
Can't say	0.01	0.01	0.01	0.01	0.01	0.00	0.01	0.01	0.01
Current health compared with health six months ago									
Much better	0.05	0.05	0.05	0.04	0.02	0.10	0.05	0.05	0.05
Somewhat better	0.07	0.07	0.08	0.08	0.08	0.08	0.07	0.07	0.08
Same	0.73	0.72	0.74	0.77	0.78	0.74	0.73	0.72	0.74
Somewhat worse	0.12	0.13	0.10	0.07	0.07	0.08	0.12	0.13	0.10
Much worse	0.02	0.02	0.02	0.04	0.05	0.00	0.02	0.02	0.02
Can't say	0.01	0.01	0.00	0.01	0.01	0.00	0.01	0.01	0.00
Expected health status six months from now									
Better	0.10	0.08	0.12	0.12	0.11	0.15	0.10	0.08	0.12
Same	0.66	0.64	0.68	0.71	0.69	0.79	0.66	0.64	0.68
Worse	0.07	0.09	0.04	0.05	0.06	0.03	0.07	0.09	0.04
Can't say	0.18	0.19	0.16	0.12	0.15	0.03	0.18	0.19	0.16
Serious illness in past year	0.32	0.34	0.31	0.35	0.31	0.38	0.32	0.34	0.31
Social activities limited by health									
None	0.66	0.64	0.68	0.69	0.67	0.77	0.66	0.64	0.68
Some	0.23	0.24	0.22	0.21	0.24	0.10	0.23	0.24	0.22
Most	0.07	0.08	0.06	0.08	0.08	0.08	0.07	0.08	0.06
All	0.02	0.03	0.02	0.01	0.01	0.03	0.02	0.03	0.02
Can't say	0.02	0.01	0.02	0.01	0.01	0.03	0.02	0.01	0.02

Table 5.3—Continued

	All Sponsors[a]			Enrolled Sponsors			Nonenrolled Sponsors		
	All	TX	CA	All	TX	CA	All	TX	CA
Medical conditions									
Arteriosclerosis	0.12	0.12	0.12	0.10	0.08	0.18	0.12	0.12	0.12
Hypertension	0.53	0.51	0.54	0.46	0.47	0.44	0.53	0.51	0.54
Heart attack	0.16	0.20	0.11	0.15	0.16	0.13	0.16	0.20	0.11
Coronary heart disease	0.16	0.16	0.15	0.13	0.10	0.21	0.16	0.16	0.15
Congestive heart failure	0.07	0.08	0.07	0.04	0.04	0.03	0.07	0.08	0.07
Stroke	0.08	0.09	0.07	0.04	0.04	0.03	0.08	0.09	0.07
Skin cancer	0.23	0.27	0.19	0.29	0.32	0.21	0.23	0.27	0.19
Cancer (other)	0.17	0.17	0.16	0.19	0.19	0.18	0.17	0.17	0.16
Diabetes	0.16	0.16	0.15	0.17	0.15	0.23	0.16	0.16	0.15
Arthritis	0.11	0.13	0.09	0.10	0.12	0.05	0.11	0.13	0.09
Osteoporosis	0.03	0.05	0.02	0.05	0.06	0.03	0.03	0.05	0.02
Parkinson's disease	0.01	0.01	0.01	0.01	0.01	0.00	0.01	0.01	0.01
Emphysema, asthma, chronic pulmonary obstructive disorder	0.13	0.14	0.11	0.14	0.14	0.15	0.13	0.14	0.11
Paralysis	0.01	0.02	0.01	0.04	0.03	0.05	0.01	0.02	0.01
None of above	0.15	0.14	0.16	0.18	0.17	0.23	0.15	0.14	0.16
Mean number of medical conditions	2.1	2.2	2.0	2.0	2.0	2.1	2.1	2.2	2.0
Standard deviation	*1.4*	*1.5*	*1.2*	*1.4*	*1.4*	*1.5*	*1.4*	*1.5*	*1.2*
Receive help from others with personal-care needs									
None of the time	0.90	0.90	0.90	0.95	0.94	0.95	0.90	0.90	0.90
Some of the time	0.07	0.07	0.08	0.04	0.04	0.03	0.07	0.07	0.08
Most of the time	0.02	0.02	0.01	0.01	0.02	0.00	0.02	0.02	0.01
All of the time	0.01	0.02	0.01	0.00	0.00	0.00	0.01	0.02	0.01
Can't say	0.00	0.00	0.00	0.01	0.00	0.03	0.00	0.00	0.00

Table 5.3—Continued

	All Sponsors[a]			Enrolled Sponsors			Nonenrolled Sponsors		
	All	TX	CA	All	TX	CA	All	TX	CA
Amount of care received at MTFs									
None	0.89	0.88	0.90	0.94	0.94	0.92	0.89	0.88	0.90
Some	0.07	0.07	0.01	0.04	0.03	0.08	0.07	0.07	0.01
Most	0.02	0.02	0.02	0.02	0.02	0.00	0.02	0.02	0.02
All	0.01	0.02	0.01	0.00	0.00	0.00	0.01	0.02	0.01
Don't know	0.00	0.00	0.00	0.00	0.00	0.00	0.00	0.00	0.00
Where most prescriptions are filled									
Military pharmacy/mail order	0.25	0.32	0.18	0.41	0.41	0.40	0.24	0.31	0.18
Civilian pharmacy/mail order	0.57	0.52	0.63	0.55	0.55	0.55	0.57	0.52	0.63
VA pharmacy/mail order	0.18	0.22	0.12	0.14	0.15	0.13	0.18	0.23	0.12
Other	0.12	0.07	0.18	0.09	0.11	0.05	0.12	0.07	0.18
Don't know	0.00	0.00	0.00	0.00	0.00	0.00	0.00	0.00	0.00

[a]Weighted to reflect differential probability of sampling for enrollees and nonenrollees.

Approximately one-quarter of sponsors reported having been hospitalized in the previous year and slightly more reported having used an emergency room in that period. Neither the hospitalization nor emergency-room usage rate varied substantially by TSSD enrollment status, nor did the mean number of physician visits or prescriptions used in the past year vary substantially by TSSD enrollment status. (Surprisingly, despite the different rates of drug coverage, the mean number of prescription drugs also did not differ substantially by study site.)

In terms of health status, enrolled sponsors reported themselves being in better general health than did nonenrolled sponsors; however, similar patterns were not observed for prior and expected future health, serious illness in the past year, social limitations, or the prevalence of illness. Enrollees were somewhat more likely to report receiving help from others (which may be because more enrollees than nonenrollees are married and thus more enrollees have a spouse available to help them).

Finally, enrollees were slightly less likely than nonenrollees to have received medical care at MTFs in the year preceding the survey and were substantially more likely than nonenrollees in both Texas and California to fill prescriptions using military pharmacies. However, both of these patterns may be artifacts of TSSD participation, which locks enrollees out of MTFs but gives them access to the TSSD (military-sponsored) pharmacy benefit.

Health insurance, health care usage, and health-status patterns for spouses (see Table 5.4) were generally similar to those for sponsors. In particular, enrolled spouses reported substantially better self-rated health than did nonenrolled spouses.

Health Insurance Preferences

Table 5.5 presents sponsors' self-reported preferences for particular health insurance characteristics by TSSD enrollment status and state of residence. The far-left column of the table lists beneficiaries' reports of the health plan features they find most essential. Low out-of-pocket costs for hospital care (reported by 72 percent), low out-of-pocket costs for prescriptions (reported by 71 percent), and choice of physician (reported by 59 percent) are most likely to be rated as "must haves." When asked to focus on two factors that were most important to them, respondents most consistently identified low out-of-pocket costs for hospital care and prescription drugs (each identified by 18 percent of respondents), followed by low monthly premiums (cited by 17 percent) and choice of doctor (cited by 16

Table 5.4

Spouses' Health Insurance, Health Care Usage, and Health Status

	All Spouses[a]			Enrolled Spouses			Nonenrolled Spouses		
	All	TX	CA	All	TX	CA	All	TX	CA
N (sample size)	761	412	349	110	82	28	651	330	321
Current health insurance									
Medicare or Medicare+Public	—	—	—	—	—	—	0.20	0.12	0.29
Private supplemental or HMO	—	—	—	—	—	—	0.54	0.60	0.48
Employer sponsored	—	—	—	—	—	—	0.26	0.28	0.23
TSSD	—	—	—	1.00	1.00	1.00	—	—	—
Any hospital stay in past year	0.20	0.21	0.19	0.20	0.23	0.07	0.21	0.23	0.19
Any emergency room visit in past year	0.28	0.25	0.30	0.25	0.31	0.08	0.29	0.27	0.31
Mean number of physician visits in past year	6.6	6.5	6.6	6.6	6.6	6.4	6.9	7.0	6.8
Standard deviation	4.2	4.1	4.3	3.9	3.9	3.9	4.4	4.4	4.4
Mean number of prescription medications	4.0	4.3	3.8	3.9	4.0	3.3	4.2	4.6	3.9
Standard deviation	2.2	2.1	2.1	2.2	2.2	2.2	2.3	2.3	2.2
General health status									
Excellent	0.09	0.07	0.10	0.20	0.20	0.20	0.09	0.07	0.10
Very good	0.24	0.21	0.28	0.28	0.25	0.40	0.25	0.22	0.29
Good	0.33	0.34	0.33	0.28	0.27	0.32	0.35	0.36	0.34
Fair	0.20	0.21	0.19	0.16	0.19	0.08	0.21	0.22	0.19
Poor	0.09	0.10	0.07	0.08	0.10	0.00	0.09	0.11	0.07
Can't say	0.01	0.01	0.01	0.00	0.00	0.00	0.01	0.01	0.01

Table 5.4—Continued

	All Spouses[a]			Enrolled Spouses			Nonenrolled Spouses		
	All	TX	CA	All	TX	CA	All	TX	CA
Current health compared with health six months ago									
Much better	0.03	0.03	0.04	0.06	0.04	0.12	0.03	0.03	0.04
Somewhat better	0.07	0.06	0.09	0.07	0.05	0.12	0.07	0.06	0.09
Same	0.72	0.71	0.73	0.74	0.74	0.72	0.75	0.76	0.75
Somewhat worse	0.11	0.11	0.11	0.14	0.17	0.04	0.12	0.12	0.11
Much worse	0.01	0.02	0.01	0.00	0.00	0.00	0.01	0.02	0.01
Can't say	0.00	0.01	0.00	0.00	0.00	0.00	0.00	0.01	0.00
Serious illness in past year	0.27	0.28	0.25	0.27	0.29	0.20	0.28	0.30	0.26
Receive help from others									
None	0.85	0.83	0.87	0.86	0.84	0.92	0.89	0.89	0.89
Some	0.07	0.07	0.07	0.10	0.13	0.00	0.07	0.07	0.07
Most	0.02	0.02	0.02	0.04	0.02	0.80	0.02	0.02	0.02
All	0.02	0.03	0.02	0.00	0.00	0.00	0.02	0.03	0.02
Can't say	0.00	0.00	0.00	0.00	0.00	0.00	0.00	0.00	0.00
Amount of care received at MTFs									
None	0.91	0.90	0.93	0.98	0.98	1.00	0.95	0.96	0.95
Some	0.03	0.03	0.03	0.01	0.01	0.00	0.03	0.03	0.03
Most	0.01	0.01	0.01	0.00	0.00	0.00	0.01	0.01	0.01
All	0.00	0.00	0.00	0.00	0.00	0.00	0.00	0.00	0.00
Don't know	0.00	0.00	0.01	0.01	0.01	0.00	0.00	0.00	0.01

NOTE: The sample frame for spouses consists of eligible spouses married to an eligible sponsor, with the sponsor living in the household.

[a]Weighted to reflect differential probability of sampling for enrollees and nonenrollees.

Table 5.5

Sponsors' Health Insurance Preferences: Essential and Nonessential Characteristics

	All Sponsors[a]			Enrolled Sponsors			Nonenrolled Sponsors		
	All	TX	CA	All	TX	CA	All	TX	CA
N (sample size)	1,180	641	539	168	128	40	1,012	513	499
"Must Have" insurance characteristics									
Low monthly premiums	0.55	0.60	0.50	0.53	0.54	0.50	0.55	0.60	0.50
Coverage outside United States	0.09	0.04	0.14	0.07	0.04	0.15	0.09	0.04	0.14
Low out-of-pocket costs for physician visits	0.58	0.62	0.55	0.55	0.55	0.55	0.58	0.62	0.55
Low out-of-pocket costs for hospital visits	0.72	0.73	0.70	0.75	0.75	0.75	0.72	0.73	0.70
Coverage for preventive services	0.51	0.51	0.51	0.48	0.48	0.48	0.51	0.51	0.51
Choice of physician	0.59	0.65	0.53	0.64	0.61	0.75	0.59	0.65	0.52
Choice of hospital	0.52	0.61	0.43	0.55	0.52	0.65	0.52	0.62	0.42
Coverage for mental health	0.19	0.19	0.18	0.17	0.20	0.10	0.19	0.19	0.18
Minimal paperwork	0.33	0.33	0.32	0.32	0.31	0.35	0.33	0.33	0.32
Low out-of-pocket costs for drugs	0.71	0.74	0.68	0.76	0.75	0.78	0.71	0.74	0.68
Being able to keep current physician	0.50	0.58	0.43	0.60	0.58	0.65	0.50	0.58	0.42

Table 5.5—Continued

	All Sponsors[a]			Enrolled Sponsors			Nonenrolled Sponsors		
	All	TX	CA	All	TX	CA	All	TX	CA
"Don't Need" insurance characteristics									
Low monthly premiums	0.05	0.04	0.06	0.03	0.03	0.03	0.05	0.04	0.06
Coverage outside United States	0.55	0.65	0.43	0.58	0.62	0.48	0.55	0.65	0.43
Low out-of-pocket costs for physician visits	0.04	0.04	0.04	0.02	0.02	0.05	0.04	0.04	0.04
Low out-of-pocket costs for hospital visits	0.05	0.04	0.05	0.01	0.01	0.03	0.05	0.04	0.05
Coverage for preventive services	0.06	0.06	0.07	0.04	0.04	0.05	0.06	0.06	0.07
Choice of physician	0.03	0.03	0.04	0.03	0.02	0.05	0.03	0.03	0.04
Choice of hospital	0.04	0.02	0.06	0.02	0.02	0.03	0.04	0.02	0.06
Coverage for mental health	0.34	0.34	0.34	0.39	0.39	0.40	0.34	0.34	0.34
Minimal paperwork	0.10	0.09	0.12	0.03	0.03	0.03	0.10	0.09	0.12
Low out-of-pocket costs for drugs	0.04	0.03	0.04	0.01	0.01	0.00	0.04	0.03	0.04
Being able to keep current physician	0.07	0.04	0.09	0.03	0.02	0.05	0.07	0.04	0.09

[a]Weighted to reflect differential probability of sampling for enrollees and nonenrollees.

percent). Somewhat surprisingly, low out-of-pocket costs for office visits were emphasized less frequently.

We also asked respondents to identify the characteristics they found to be nonessential. The only characteristics that more than 20 percent of all respondents identified as *not* being necessary were coverage outside the United States and coverage for mental health care. Those two characteristics, along with minimal paperwork, were also those most frequently identified when beneficiaries were asked to identify two characteristics that were least important to them.

Attitudes Toward Military Health Care

Table 5.6 reports the results of respondents being asked to indicate their agreement or disagreement with five statements about military health benefits. Twice as many beneficiaries disagreed as agreed with the statement, "Military retirees and their dependents can count on getting care at MTFs when they need it." An overwhelming majority of respondents agreed that retirees over 65 and their dependents should have the option of enrolling in TRICARE. Four times as many disagreed as agreed with statements that retirees should contribute to the cost of their health care and that health benefits for military retirees aged 65 and over were generous, relative to other employers. Finally, nearly half agreed that they preferred military-sponsored health care, assuming cost was not an issue.

Knowledge of TSSD and Attitudes Regarding Enrollment

We asked beneficiaries about how they gained their knowledge of TSSD (the results are shown in Table 5.7). Not surprisingly, all enrolled sponsors reported having been aware of the demonstration prior to receiving the survey. However, only half of nonenrollees reported that they had previously heard of the demonstration.

Among those who knew about the demonstration, their main sources of information were similar. Three-fourths of knowledgeable beneficiaries reported reading materials provided by the military (i.e., materials from TMA). Slightly fewer than half reported receiving materials from retiree organizations; as we noted earlier, enrollees were substantially more likely to belong to an association of military retirees. About 15 percent of enrollees, but only 3 percent of nonenrollees, reported having attended a town meeting about TSSD.

Table 5.6

Sponsors' Attitudes Toward Military Health Care

	All Sponsors[a]			Enrolled Sponsors			Nonenrolled Sponsors		
	All	TX	CA	All	TX	CA	All	TX	CA
N (sample size)	1,180	641	539	168	128	40	1,012	513	499
Agree or strongly agree									
Can count on care at MTFs	0.27	0.23	0.29	0.17	0.15	0.25	0.27	0.24	0.29
Should have option to enroll in TRICARE	0.84	0.87	0.81	0.95	0.95	0.95	0.83	0.86	0.81
Should contribute to cost of own health care	0.16	0.13	0.18	0.20	0.20	0.20	0.16	0.13	0.18
Military offers good retiree benefits	0.14	0.13	0.14	0.20	0.19	0.25	0.14	0.13	0.14
Prefer military-sponsored health care over other health-care options	0.42	0.45	0.38	0.49	0.48	0.53	0.42	0.45	0.38
Disagree or strongly disagree									
Can count on care at MTFs	0.50	0.54	0.47	0.54	0.56	0.48	0.50	0.54	0.47
Should have option to enroll in TRICARE	0.02	0.02	0.01	0.02	0.02	0.00	0.02	0.02	0.01
Should contribute to cost of own health care	0.62	0.70	0.53	0.63	0.64	0.60	0.62	0.70	0.53
Military offers good retiree benefits	0.61	0.64	0.57	0.55	0.57	0.48	0.61	0.65	0.57
Prefer military-sponsored health care over other health-care options	0.22	0.25	0.19	0.22	0.23	0.18	0.22	0.25	0.19

[a]Weighted to reflect differential probability of sampling for enrollees and nonenrollees.

Table 5.7

How Sponsors Gained Knowledge About TSSD

	All Sponsors[a]			Enrolled Sponsors			Nonenrolled Sponsors		
	All	TX	CA	All	TX	CA	All	TX	CA
N (sample size)	1,180	641	539	168	128	40	1,012	513	499
Already knew about TSSD	0.52	0.52	0.53	0.99	0.98	1.00	0.50	0.49	0.52
Source of information about TSSD									
Read information from military	0.75	0.70	0.80	0.71	0.71	0.70	0.75	0.70	0.80
Received information from retiree organization	0.44	0.43	0.46	0.42	0.41	0.45	0.44	0.43	0.46
From congressperson	0.01	0.02	0.00	0.01	0.01	0.00	0.01	0.02	0.00
Health fair/town meeting	0.04	0.04	0.03	0.14	0.15	0.13	0.03	0.03	0.03
Radio/television	0.01	0.01	0.00	0.01	0.01	0.00	0.01	0.01	0.00
Local newspaper	0.05	0.05	0.04	0.02	0.03	0.00	0.05	0.05	0.04
Family/friends	0.06	0.07	0.04	0.04	0.06	0.00	0.06	0.07	0.04
Other	0.08	0.08	0.07	0.13	0.14	0.10	0.07	0.07	0.07
Not sure	0.02	0.02	0.03	0.02	0.02	0.00	0.02	0.02	0.03

[a]Weighted to reflect differential probability of sampling for enrollees and nonenrollees.

Only one-fifth of enrollees reported that they had difficulty deciding whether to enroll in TSSD (see Table 5.8). The table shows that their main source of uncertainty had to do with their concern about dropping other supplemental coverage. The fraction was lower in California, perhaps due to the prevalence of Medicare HMOs and because Medicare rules preclude medical underwriting and guarantee all eligible beneficiaries access to all such plans that are available in a particular area. However, California enrollees were relatively more worried than were Texas enrollees about paperwork burdens; this may be due to their prior experience with Medicare HMOs, which require relatively little paperwork. Other major concerns for enrollees related to how TSSD would be integrated with Medicare, uncertainty about the benefit structure, and concerns about provider access.

Nonenrollees (who knew about TSSD) were more than twice as likely as enrollees to report having difficulty deciding whether to enroll. Like the enrollees, the majority of nonenrollees were concerned about dropping other Medigap coverage. Other areas of concern for nonenrollees included uncertainty about costs as well as the other issues emphasized by enrollees.

Stated Reasons for Enrollment or Nonenrollment

We asked nonenrollees to report the reasons why they did not enroll in TSSD (see Table 5.9), and we asked enrollees to report their reasons for enrolling (see Table 5.10). Nonenrolled sponsors emphasized two factors: (1) They were satisfied with their current plan, particularly in California, and (2) they didn't receive enough information about TSSD to make a decision. Another main factor they identified was their desire to avoid burdensome paperwork.

Among enrollees, the most important determinants included lower costs (identified as a factor by more than 80 percent of enrollees and identified as one of the two most important determinants by half of the enrollees) and better drug coverage, particularly for beneficiaries in Texas. California beneficiaries were more likely than beneficiaries in Texas to emphasize that TSSD gave them a wide choice of providers. Overall, half of the enrollees reported being very satisfied with TSSD, and nearly 90 percent reported being somewhat or very satisfied.

Analysis of Enrollment

In the remainder of this chapter, we focus on factors associated with TSSD enrollment and health plan choice, using multivariate modeling. For models that

Table 5.8

Reasons for Difficulty Deciding Whether to Enroll, Sponsors Who Already Knew About TSSD

	All Sponsors[a]			Enrolled Sponsors			Nonenrolled Sponsors		
	All	TX	CA	All	TX	CA	All	TX	CA
N (sample size)	1,180	641	539	168	128	40	1,012	513	499
Had difficulty deciding	0.43	0.45	0.39	0.19	0.20	0.18	0.45	0.49	0.40
Reasons for difficulty in deciding									
Unsure about cost	0.55	0.48	0.65	0.16	0.21	0.00	0.57	0.50	0.66
Unsure with regard to integration with Medicare	0.56	0.52	0.61	0.39	0.38	0.43	0.57	0.53	0.61
Unsure about benefits	0.44	0.40	0.48	0.35	0.33	0.43	0.44	0.40	0.48
Unsure about available providers	0.53	0.46	0.60	0.32	0.33	0.29	0.54	0.47	0.61
Unsure about paperwork	0.33	0.29	0.38	0.32	0.25	0.57	0.33	0.29	0.38
Hard to compare to other plans	0.44	0.36	0.53	0.19	0.17	0.29	0.45	0.37	0.53
Concerned about dropping other plans	0.67	0.67	0.67	0.71	0.75	0.57	0.67	0.67	0.67
Other	0.22	0.20	0.24	0.19	0.21	0.14	0.22	0.20	0.24
Can't say	0.02	0.03	0.00	0.03	0.00	0.14	0.02	0.03	0.00

[a]Weighted to reflect differential probability of sampling for enrollees and nonenrollees.

Table 5.9

Reasons Reported by Eligible Nonenrollees for Not Enrolling in TSSD

	Nonenrolled Sponsors			Nonenrolled Spouses		
	All	TX	CA	All	TX	CA
N (sample size)	1,012	513	499	651	330	321
Reason for not enrolling						
Not eligible	0.038	0.049	0.026	0.058	0.069	0.047
Satisfied with current coverage	0.429	0.292	0.563	0.418	0.315	0.520
Plan to enroll but have not done so yet	0.126	0.144	0.108	0.089	0.112	0.065
Dislike military health care	0.053	0.038	0.067	0.067	0.054	0.079
Want benefits that are not covered	0.075	0.076	0.075	0.056	0.058	0.054
Do not like TRICARE providers	0.056	0.061	0.052	0.058	0.043	0.072
Do not like filing claims	0.284	0.242	0.325	0.208	0.185	0.231
Did not get enough information	0.466	0.481	0.451	—	—	—
Snowbird	0.034	0.042	0.026	—	—	—
Not a permanent program	0.289	0.303	0.276	—	—	—
Other	0.252	0.265	0.239	0.374	0.449	0.300
Not sure	0.100	0.106	0.093	0.116	0.112	0.119

NOTE: Not all of the questions directed to sponsors (i.e., eligible nonenrollees) were directed to the nonenrollees' spouses (the dashes indicate questions the spouses were not asked).

examine TSSD enrollment per se, we use standard (binary) logistic regression. For models that examine health plan choice (e.g., Medicare only, Medicare+private Medigap, Medicare+employer plan, TSSD), we use multinomial logistic regression. We estimate models that pool Texas and California respondents and estimate a second set of models on just the California respondents; estimation of the second set was motivated by the availability of Medicare+Choice HMOs in California but not in Texas.

In all cases, because the parameters from logistic regression are difficult to interpret directly, we present predicted enrollment rates, standardized for all the other characteristics included in a particular model. The following tables present the marginal effects on enrollment rates of each covariate included in that particular model.

Due to the nature of our survey data, we did not control for certain characteristics that might be expected to influence health plan choice. For instance, we expected that beneficiaries with poor knowledge of TSSD would be relatively less likely to enroll and that beneficiaries who used a lot of prescription drugs would find TSSD relatively attractive. However, our survey data were

60

Table 5.10

Enrollees' Reasons for Enrolling in TSSD and Level of Satisfaction with the Program

	Enrolled Sponsors			Enrolled Spouses		
	All	TX	CA	All	TX	CA
N (sample size)	168	128	40	110	82	28
Joined TSSD because						
Costs less	0.870	0.894	0.789	0.879	0.927	0.720
Good benefit package	0.801	0.805	0.789	0.766	0.793	0.680
Wide choice of providers	0.559	0.537	0.632	0.654	0.744	0.360
Better drug coverage	0.789	0.829	0.658	0.215	0.232	0.160
Good reputation for quality	0.124	0.106	0.184	0.028	0.024	0.040
Do not want to use military facilities	0.186	0.195	0.158	0.523	0.537	0.480
Friends and family recommended it	0.043	0.049	0.026	0.215	0.207	0.240
Want to be in same plan as spouse	0.329	0.341	0.289	0.028	0.024	0.040
Prefer to have military-sponsored care	0.317	0.325	0.289	0.009	0.012	0.000
Other	0.050	0.049	0.053	—	—	—
Not sure	0.012	0.016	0.000	—	—	—
Satisfaction with TSSD						
Very satisfied	0.500	0.509	0.472	0.439	0.463	0.360
Satisfied	0.375	0.397	0.306	0.449	0.451	0.440
Not satisfied	0.059	0.043	0.111	0.065	0.049	0.120
Cannot say	0.066	0.052	0.111	0.047	0.037	0.080

NOTE: Not all of the questions directed to sponsors (i.e., eligible nonenrollees) were directed to the nonenrollees' spouses (the dashes indicate questions the spouses were not asked).

collected well into the demonstration period, leading to the likelihood of reverse causality between TSSD enrollment on the one hand and characteristics such as knowledge about the program and health care use on the other. We therefore focus on characteristics that are plausibly exogenous with respect to TSSD enrollment.

Table 5.11 presents predictors of TSSD enrollment, using all survey respondents. Although the effect of age is substantively large, with younger beneficiaries more likely to enroll in TSSD, it is not statistically significant at conventional levels. The factors with a significant effect on TSSD enrollment include marital status, with married beneficiaries being more likely to enroll; income (at p<0.10), with lower-income beneficiaries being more likely to enroll; membership in a retiree organization, with members being more likely to enroll; officer status, with officers being substantially more likely to enroll; and self-rated general health, with beneficiaries in excellent or very good health being more likely to enroll. Enrollment rates were also significantly higher in Texas. In general, these patterns mirror those observed in the cross-tabulations.

Table 5.11

Predictors of TSSD Enrollment

	Predicted Fraction Enrolled	P-value of Contrast
Age 65[a]	0.061	0.136
Age 75[a]	0.049	
Age 85[a]	0.040	
Female	0.071	0.541
Male	0.050	
White	0.051	0.917
Non-white	0.049	
High school	0.047	0.386
More than high school	0.056	
Unmarried	0.032	0.040
Married	0.055	
Income $25K[a]	0.063	0.057
Income $50K[a]	0.051	
Income $75K[a]	0.042	
Belongs to retiree organization	0.059	0.016
No membership in retiree organization	0.039	
Non-officer	0.030	0.000
Officer	0.096	
No serious illness	0.047	0.199
Serious illness	0.059	
Excellent/very good health	0.058	0.015
Good/fair/poor health	0.033	
Previously had private Medigap[b]	0.045	0.137
No previous private Medigap	0.059	
Previously had employer plan[b]	0.016	0.000
No previous employer plan	0.064	
Low monthly premiums not essential	0.046	0.467
Low monthly premiums essential	0.054	
Low physician copayments not essential	0.062	0.112
Low physician copayments essential	0.044	

Table 5.11—Continued

	Predicted Fraction Enrolled	P-value of Contrast
Paperwork requirements not essential	0.053	0.538
Minimal paperwork essential	0.047	
Low prescription copays not essential	0.040	0.226
Low prescription copays essential	0.054	
No preference for military health care	0.046	0.851
Strong preference for military health care	0.051	
California	0.028	0.000
Texas	0.069	

NOTE: This table includes the predicted fraction enrolling in TSSD, standardized for the covariates in the table. The sample includes all survey respondents, excluding those whose self-reported TSSD enrollment status conflicted with DEERS and those who reported that they were not eligible for Medicare (sample number=1,124).

[a]Age and income are entered into the model as continuous variables, but their effect on enrollment is evaluated at discrete points. The p-value is for the test of the effect of the continuous variable against zero.

[b]Indicators of previous insurance in the models underlying this table *are not* mutually exclusive.

Perhaps most important from a policy perspective, beneficiaries with employer-sponsored supplemental coverage were substantially less likely to enroll in TSSD than those without such coverage.

Somewhat surprisingly, given the results shown earlier in this chapter, stated preferences for low premiums, low physician and prescription copayments, and minimal paperwork were not significantly associated with TSSD enrollment. And neither was beneficiaries' preference for military-sponsored health care significantly associated with TSSD enrollment, although the interpretation of this measure might be somewhat ambiguous: On the one hand, TSSD was a military-sponsored health plan; on the other hand, enrolling in TSSD locked beneficiaries out of MTFs.

The lack of relationship between beneficiaries' stated insurance preferences and TSSD participation may reflect their relatively poor understanding of the demonstration program. Such confusion would make it difficult for beneficiaries to make choices that are consistent with their preferences. However, there may be other explanations, including the possibility that TSSD does not differ systematically from beneficiaries' alternative choices with respect to the characteristics assessed here. (Indeed, as we report later, these characteristics also are not predictive of beneficiaries' broader health insurance choices—e.g., Medicare only, private Medigap, employer-sponsored Medigap, and TSSD).

Table 5.12 presents results analogous to those in Table 5.11 but for just the California sample. We examined these beneficiaries separately to assess the effects of the availability of Medicare+Choice HMOs in California. Indeed, beneficiaries with prior employer-sponsored coverage, or who were enrolled in a Medicare HMO, were significantly less likely to enroll than those with private or no supplemental insurance. The only other significant predictor of enrollment in the California subsample was officer status, with officers being significantly more likely to enroll.

Table 5.12

Predictors of TSSD Enrollment, California Sample Only

	Predicted Fraction Enrolled	P-value of Contrast
Age 65[a]	0.054	0.017
Age 75[a]	0.030	
Age 85[a]	0.016	
Female	0.043	0.705
Male	0.028	
White	0.029	0.623
Non-white	0.023	
High school	0.027	0.920
More than high school	0.027	
Unmarried	0.015	0.158
Married	0.032	
Income $25K[a]	0.033	0.516
Income $50K[a]	0.030	
Income $75K[a]	0.027	
Belongs to retiree organization	0.034	0.198
No membership in retiree organization	0.022	
Non-officer	0.014	0.002
Officer	0.045	
No serious illness	0.025	0.269
Serious illness	0.036	
Excellent/very good health	0.032	0.149
Good/fair/poor health	0.015	

Table 5.12—Continued

	Predicted Fraction Enrolled	P-value of Contrast
Previously had private Medigap[b]	0.053	0.000
Previously had employer Medigap[b]	0.014	
Previously had Medicare HMO[b]	0.011	
No previous supplemental plan[b]	0.077	
Low monthly premiums not essential	0.023	0.386
Low monthly premiums essential	0.033	
Low physician copayments not essential	0.030	0.711
Low physician copayments essential	0.026	
Paperwork requirements not essential	0.029	0.760
Minimal paperwork essential	0.026	
Low prescription copays not essential	0.019	0.324
Low prescription copays essential	0.031	
No preference for military health care	0.015	0.369
Strong preference for military health care	0.029	

NOTE: The table includes the predicted fraction enrolling in TSSD, standardized for the covariates in the table. The sample includes all survey respondents in California, excluding those whose self-reported TSSD enrollment status conflicted with DEERS and those who reported that they were not eligible for Medicare (sample number=505).

[a]Age and income are entered into the model as continuous variables, but their effect on enrollment is evaluated at discrete points. The p-value is for the test of the effect of the continuous variable against zero.

[b]Indicators of previous insurance in the models underlying this table *are* mutually exclusive.

It is difficult to know why relatively few factors are significantly associated with TSSD enrollment among respondents in California relative to TSSD enrollment among respondents in Texas. One factor may be the smaller number of enrollees in California, which in turn may be due to the availability of Medicare+Choice HMOs in California but not in Texas.

Table 5.13 presents results of multinomial models of health insurance choice. The table presents the estimated distribution of enrollment across the various plan choices, standardizing for the other characteristics in the model, which are presented in the table.

The characteristics with a large substantive effect include age, with higher age increasing the probability that the beneficiary has only Medicare; gender, with women being substantially less likely to have private supplemental coverage and more likely to have employer-sponsored coverage (note that the sample contains very few female sponsors); income, with higher-income respondents less likely to have private Medigap and substantially more likely to have employer-sponsored

Table 5.13

Predictors of Current Health Plan Choice

	Medicare Only	Medicare + Private Plan	Medicare + Employer Plan	TSSD	P-Value of Contrast
Age 65[a]	0.201	0.461	0.279	0.059	0.143
Age 75[a]	0.245	0.452	0.257	0.047	
Age 85[a]	0.294	0.436	0.234	0.036	
Female	0.243	0.317	0.374	0.065	0.700
Male	0.240	0.455	0.258	0.047	
White	0.235	0.450	0.267	0.048	0.667
Non-white	0.275	0.463	0.216	0.047	
High school	0.244	0.465	0.247	0.045	0.637
More than high school	0.230	0.431	0.285	0.053	
Unmarried	0.239	0.517	0.211	0.033	0.088
Married	0.241	0.438	0.270	0.051	
Income $25K[a]	0.252	0.497	0.189	0.062	0.000
Income $50K[a]	0.239	0.458	0.253	0.050	
Income $75K[a]	0.220	0.412	0.329	0.039	
California	0.188	0.499	0.289	0.023	0.000
Texas	0.284	0.413	0.232	0.071	
Belongs to retiree organization	0.206	0.488	0.251	0.055	0.008
No membership in retiree organization	0.274	0.417	0.270	0.039	
Non-officer	0.256	0.431	0.285	0.029	0.000
Officer	0.202	0.481	0.226	0.090	
No serious illness	0.231	0.467	0.258	0.044	0.450
Serious illness	0.257	0.424	0.264	0.056	
Excellent/very good health	0.252	0.454	0.263	0.032	0.115
Good/fair/poor health	0.235	0.452	0.259	0.055	
Low monthly premiums not essential	0.233	0.474	0.247	0.046	0.872
Low monthly premiums essential	0.244	0.438	0.269	0.049	

Table 5.13—Continued

	Medicare Only	Medicare + Private Plan	Medicare + Employer Plan	TSSD	P-Value of Contrast
Low physician copayments not essential	0.211	0.484	0.244	0.060	0.198
Low physician copayments essential	0.255	0.434	0.269	0.042	
Paperwork requirements not essential	0.243	0.429	0.279	0.049	0.299
Minimal paperwork essential	0.234	0.492	0.227	0.046	
Low prescription copays not essential	0.294	0.416	0.253	0.037	0.274
Low prescription copays essential	0.226	0.462	0.261	0.052	
No preference for military health care	0.786	0.125	0.027	0.063	0.000
Strong preference for military health care	0.215	0.466	0.272	0.047	

NOTE: This table includes the predicted fraction enrolling in the respective insurance options, standardized for the covariates in the table (based on a multinomial logit model). The sample includes all survey respondents, excluding those whose self-reported TSSD enrollment status conflicted with DEERS and those who reported that they were not eligible for Medicare (sample number=1,124).

[a]Age and income are entered into the model as continuous variables, but their effect on enrollment is evaluated at discrete points. The p-value is for the test of the effect of the continuous variable against zero.

coverage; state of residence, with respondents in Texas more likely to have only Medicare coverage and more likely to enroll in TSSD; membership in a military retiree organization, with members being more likely to have private Medigap; and officer status at retirement, with officers significantly more likely to have private Medigap or TSSD and less likely to have employer-sponsored insurance or Medicare only. Of these factors, the effects of age and gender are not statistically significant (at $p<0.10$) across the four outcome choices.

As in the previous models presented in this chapter, with the exception of preference for military-sponsored care, beneficiaries' insurance preferences are not significantly associated with plan choice; beneficiaries without such a preference are very likely to have only Medicare. The effects of beneficiaries' health are also not statistically significant in this model.

Finally, Table 5.14 repeats the analysis shown in Table 5.13 but for just the California sample. In this case, the model accounts for the availability of

Table 5.14

Predictors of Current Health Plan Choice, California Sample Only

	Medicare Only	Medicare+ Private	Medicare HMO	Medicare+ Employer	TSSD	P-Value
Age 65[a]	0.099	0.075	0.480	0.309	0.038	0.013
Age 75[a]	0.176	0.100	0.390	0.309	0.025	
Age 85[a]	0.292	0.123	0.288	0.283	0.015	
White	0.180	0.110	0.370	0.315	0.025	0.485
Non-white	0.217	0.068	0.431	0.265	0.019	
High school	0.191	0.094	0.400	0.290	0.025	0.974
More than high school	0.182	0.109	0.373	0.313	0.023	
Unmarried	0.191	0.132	0.379	0.283	0.015	0.640
Married	0.186	0.094	0.386	0.308	0.027	
Income $25K[a]	0.208	0.092	0.461	0.215	0.024	0.076
Income $50K[a]	0.194	0.100	0.406	0.275	0.025	
Income $75K[a]	0.178	0.107	0.349	0.342	0.025	
Belongs to retiree organization	0.169	0.111	0.380	0.316	0.024	0.814
No membership in retiree organization	0.207	0.092	0.389	0.287	0.024	
Non-officer	0.186	0.085	0.395	0.322	0.012	0.095
Officer	0.188	0.116	0.371	0.287	0.038	
No serious illness	0.191	0.078	0.410	0.301	0.021	0.106
Serious illness	0.179	0.153	0.327	0.309	0.032	
Excellent/very good health	0.165	0.096	0.432	0.292	0.015	0.673
Good/fair/poor health	0.193	0.103	0.372	0.305	0.027	
Low monthly premiums not essential	0.224	0.110	0.373	0.269	0.025	0.571
Low monthly premiums essential	0.159	0.094	0.390	0.334	0.024	
Low physician copayments not essential	0.143	0.110	0.444	0.279	0.025	0.333
Low physician copayments essential	0.224	0.094	0.347	0.312	0.023	
Paperwork requirements not essential	0.195	0.070	0.387	0.325	0.024	0.080
Minimal paperwork essential	0.172	0.162	0.377	0.265	0.024	

Table 5.14—Continued

	Medicare Only	Medicare+ Private	Medicare HMO	Medicare+ Employer	TSSD	P-Value
Low prescription copays not essential	0.219	0.100	0.315	0.349	0.017	0.504
Low prescription copays essential	0.176	0.102	0.407	0.288	0.027	
No preference for military health care	0.879	0.000	0.083	0.000	0.038	0.001
Strong preference for military health care	0.145	0.111	0.376	0.346	0.022	

NOTE: This table includes the predicted fraction enrolling in the respective insurance options, standardized for the covariates in the table (based on a multinomial logit model). The sample includes all survey respondents in California, excluding those whose self-reported TSSD enrollment status conflicted with DEERS and those who reported that they were not eligible for Medicare (sample number=1,124).

[a]Age and income are entered into the model as continuous variables, but their effect on enrollment is evaluated at discrete points. The p-value is for the test of the effect of the continuous variable against zero.

Medicare HMOs in addition to the other choices. Age again is significantly associated with plan choice, with older beneficiaries more likely to have Medicare only and less likely to have Medicare HMO coverage. Lower-income beneficiaries are significantly (at $p<0.10$) more likely to have HMO coverage and less likely to have employer-sponsored coverage. Beneficiaries in good health are somewhat more likely to have HMO coverage, but the effects of health on the distribution of outcomes do not reach statistical significance at conventional levels. Surprisingly, beneficiaries who value minimal paperwork are no more likely to have HMO coverage than those who do not value minimal paperwork but they are twice as likely to have private Medigap coverage. Finally, beneficiaries with no preference for military health care are much more likely to have Medicare only and less likely to have an HMO or employer-sponsored plan.

Comments from Respondents

The beneficiary survey invited respondents to provide comments on "anything else" that they would like to share with us. A substantial number of respondents did just that. Comments pertaining to policy issues are in Appendix F; they have been edited to preserve respondent confidentiality.

While the volume of comments was quite large, respondents concentrated on a handful of specific issues. Those issues included the following:

Provider Access

Many beneficiaries commented on the lack of access to MTF care; in some cases, it appeared that nonenrollees viewed this as a reason for not enrolling in TSSD. More generally, both enrollees and nonenrollees commented about the relative lack of access to TRICARE (network) providers, that some providers wouldn't accept TRICARE, and that beneficiaries should have a free choice of providers. We found these comments, and the parallel comments expressed by focus group participants, somewhat surprising because TSSD permitted beneficiaries to receive care from any Medicare provider (regardless of whether the providers "accepted" TRICARE) and because the financial impact to beneficiaries of using TRICARE network versus nonxtra) or from an authorized nonnetwork providers was likely to be small in general. On the other hand, beneficiaries would need to use network providers to maximize their TSSD benefit and to avoid having to file claims. Furthermore, TSSD beneficiaries would typically find it difficult to assess the out-of-pocket costs associated with using nonnetwork providers in advance because they would need to know the provider's billed charges, the Medicare allowable charge, and the TRICARE allowable charge.[2]

Claims Processing

Nonenrollees expressed concern that they would have difficulty dealing with claims processing, and indeed enrollees complained about their experience with TSSD's claims processing. In some cases, enrollees provided very detailed histories of their interaction with TSSD, which we had to edit or remove to preserve confidentiality. In general, these beneficiaries were frustrated about the length of the process, the required number of steps, and, in some cases, the outcome. These comments are consistent with TMA's acknowledged difficulty in managing the TSSD benefit and processing claims.

Costs and Coverage

Beneficiaries emphasized three issues in this area. One issue concerned prescription drug benefits—beneficiaries commented on the high costs of prescription drugs and drug coverage and on the fact that MTF pharmacies did not carry all prescription drugs. Another key issue had to do with Medicare Part

---

[2]In general, similar issues exist for out-of-network care in most preferred-provider insurance plans. To assess out-of-pocket costs in advance, beneficiaries need to know the provider's billed charges and what the plan regards as the "usual and customary" charge (because beneficiaries are generally responsible for the full cost above usual and customary). This issue is relatively important when network providers are scarce or when beneficiaries prefer nonnetwork providers.

B participation. Some beneficiaries indicated that they had not enrolled in Part B at age 65 and now had to pay substantial penalties to enroll in Part B in order to participate in TSSD. Some indicated that the penalties had precluded their enrollment in TSSD. This is also an issue for TFL, which also requires participation in Part B. A third major issue, emphasized mainly by nonenrollees, was the temporary nature of the demonstration program.

Information

Some enrollees, and many nonenrollees, commented that they did not fully understand TSSD. Furthermore, many nonenrollees stated that they had never heard of TSSD prior to our survey. These comments were also very consistent with those made by focus group participants.

Alternative Insurance

Many nonenrollees indicated that they were satisfied with their current coverage, most commonly an employer-sponsored plan or a Medicare HMO. These comments were also consistent with those made by focus group participants.

"The Promise"

The most frequent comment, from both enrollees and nonenrollees, pertained to the feeling that military beneficiaries had been promised free lifetime medical care as an inducement to enlist and continue to serve in the military and that this promise had been broken.

6. Discussion and Conclusions

As we noted earlier in this report, the DoD has a Congressional mandate to evaluate TSSD and make recommendations about its suitability as a permanent national program. The mandated evaluation was to include:

1. An analysis of the costs of the demonstration project to the United States and to the eligible individuals who participate in such a demonstration project

2. An assessment of the extent to which the demonstration project satisfies the requirements of such eligible individuals for the health care services available under the demonstration project

3. An assessment of the effect, if any, of the demonstration project on military medical readiness

4. A description of the rate of enrollment in the demonstration project of the individuals who were eligible to enroll in the demonstration project

5. An assessment of whether the demonstration project provides the most suitable model for a program to provide adequate health care services to the population consisting of eligible individuals

6. An evaluation of any other matters that the Secretary of Defense considers appropriate.

We address each of these points in turn in this chapter.

Cost of the Demonstration Project

For most beneficiaries who lacked Medicare supplemental coverage, or who were paying for private Medigap coverage, the TSSD benefit had the potential to substantially reduce their out-of-pocket costs for medical care and significantly reduce the risk of catastrophic out-of-pocket costs, relative to the status quo. Because there was no meaningful way for us to assess the empirical effect of TSSD on health care costs (due to the very low enrollment), this conclusion about cost is based on our assessment of the actuarial value of the benefit in relation to its cost and the fact that enrollees overwhelmingly identified lower costs, good benefits, and prescription drug coverage as reasons for enrollment. TSSD represented a substantially more-generous benefit than any of the standard Medigap policies (particularly regarding prescription drugs), with generally lower monthly premiums, guaranteed access for beneficiaries, and no medical underwriting.

At the same time, the relative benefits of TSSD would be reduced somewhat for beneficiaries who lack access to TRICARE network providers, both because the level of coverage is lower for nonnetwork providers and because many network providers would require TSSD beneficiaries to file claims for reimbursement. We found some geographic differences within and between the two TSSD demonstration sites in the availability of TRICARE network providers.

We note that TSSD included some cost-sharing by beneficiaries, which TFL does not. Cost-sharing has become a nearly universal feature of preretirement health insurance and of employer-sponsored Medicare supplements because it gives beneficiaries a financial incentive to reduce their health care use. The absence of cost-sharing provisions in TFL is likely to increase health care use and costs, relative to a program with modest cost-sharing, such as TSSD.

The evaluation plan did not call for measuring the costs of developing, implementing, and administering the demonstration program.

Suitability of Benefit Design

If properly administered, TSSD seemed to be appropriate for meeting the supplemental health insurance needs of Medicare-eligible military beneficiaries. As with our findings regarding TSSD costs, this conclusion is based on our assessment of the actuarial value of the benefit and on beneficiaries' comments. Despite the limitations of the program, and the fact that the demonstration program seems to have never overcome the administrative hurdles associated with its start-up, 88 percent of enrollees identified themselves as "very satisfied" or "satisfied" with TSSD (although a substantial fraction of these were in the latter category).

In addition to the administrative problems identified by TMA, there appeared to be unresolved confusion about the program among beneficiaries. Both the administrative problems and the confusion are likely to have inhibited enrollment and frustrated enrollees. In addition, several features distinguish TSSD from TFL, the permanent national program introduced to meet the health insurance needs of this beneficiary population; in general, these distinguishing features made TSSD relatively less attractive than TFL for beneficiaries and may also have inhibited enrollment in TSSD. For instance, TSSD required a monthly premium, which TFL does not, and in many circumstances, TSSD beneficiaries needed to file claims for reimbursement, whereas TFL claims are processed automatically.

TSSD also included modest cost-sharing by beneficiaries, whereas TFL eliminates virtually all cost-sharing. While modest cost-sharing can improve the efficiency of a health insurance program by giving beneficiaries a financial incentive to reduce their health care use (and particularly the use of relatively low-value services), in practice TSSD's cost-sharing rules were not transparent to beneficiaries. In particular, beneficiaries receiving care from providers outside the TRICARE network would need to know the provider's billed charges, the Medicare allowable charge, and the TRICARE allowable charge in order to calculate their out-of-pocket costs. In this sense, TSSD's design was unlikely to be efficient.

One feature TSSD and TFL have in common is the requirement that beneficiaries be enrolled in Medicare Part B. For elderly beneficiaries who may have opted out of Part B with the expectation that they would use MTF care, and in any case did so without knowing that Part B participation would subsequently be required for access to TSSD or TFL, the financial penalty associated with enrolling now may present an economic hardship. In practice, this penalty seems to have inhibited TSSD enrollment.

Military Medical Readiness

TSSD as a demonstration program is unlikely to have had any effect on military medical readiness. By design, it was conducted outside of any MTF catchment area. That factor, plus the low enrollment, suggests that the military health care delivery system is unlikely to have been affected by TSSD in any substantive way.

As a national policy, TSSD could have affected medical readiness primarily by affecting the type and number of Medicare-eligible military beneficiaries seeking care at MTFs. However, given the scope and outcomes of the demonstration, there was no way to assess this issue definitively with respect to TSSD.

We note that possible diversion of elderly patients away from MTFs is also an issue for TFL, which, unlike TSSD, does not preclude beneficiaries from receiving care at MTFs, but which seems likely to reduce the relative attractiveness of MTF care for beneficiaries. Concern about this issue underlies the DoD's recent introduction of TRICARE Plus, a program that is intended to facilitate a stable flow of elderly patients to MTFs by giving some Medicare-eligible military beneficiaries priority access to MTF primary-care providers.[1] A broader discussion of the role that Medicare-eligible patients play in military medical readiness is outside the scope of this project.

Enrollment Rate

We have described the very low TSSD enrollment-rate patterns earlier in this report. Because of this outcome of the demonstration, a main focus of this evaluation was on the question of why enrollment rates were so low. A number of factors likely contributed to this outcome. One such factor is poor awareness and lack of understanding of the program. Half of the nonenrollees claimed not to have heard of TSSD prior to our survey. And focus group participants and survey respondents indicated that they confused TSSD with TRICARE Prime, where care is often provided at MTFs in many cases, so some identified their lack of proximity to an MTF as a reason for not enrolling. Some survey respondents indicated that they confused TSSD with TFL (for which they had just become eligible on October 1, 2001). One explanation for our finding that members of military retiree organizations were significantly more likely than other respondents to enroll in TSSD was that those organizations help disseminate information about the program.

Even among those who had heard of TSSD, a substantial fraction indicated that they were confused about the benefit design. Indeed, the benefit design was somewhat complex, particularly in the case of care received from providers outside the TRICARE network. Partly as a result of this confusion over the benefit design, beneficiaries seemed focused on the availability and quality of TRICARE network providers even though, in our view, the level of concern about provider availability and quality was out of proportion to the relative financial cost of using nonnetwork providers under TSSD. The focus on TSSD network providers may also have reflected a strong preference for avoiding claims paperwork and balance billing, which would further inhibit enrollment.

Another factor inhibiting enrollment may have been the cost of the program. Despite our assessment of the relatively high actuarial value of the TSSD benefit, beneficiaries (in both the survey and in open-ended comments) identified the program's costs as a reason for nonparticipation. It seems plausible that beneficiaries with employer-sponsored insurance or a generous

---

[1] For additional information on TRICARE Plus, see http://www.tricare.osd.mil/ Plus/default.htm.

Medicare+Choice HMO plan would have faced higher costs under TSSD. In addition, some poorer beneficiaries may have felt unable to bear the cost of the TSSD premium. Although overall enrollment rates were low, higher-income beneficiaries were significantly more likely to enroll. This is particularly true for beneficiaries who also would have faced a penalty in their Part B premium.

In our view, however, the most important factor affecting enrollment was the temporary nature of the demonstration. This issue was highlighted in our focus groups and by survey respondents. Beneficiaries with private or employer-sponsored supplemental coverage who considered enrolling in TSSD faced having to choose between paying two sets of premiums (and thus guaranteeing their access to their non-TSSD coverage if they chose to disenroll from TSSD or when the demonstration ended) or giving up their non-TSSD coverage and risking the possibility that they would have inferior supplemental coverage after TSSD. We note that beneficiaries in Medicare HMOs were less likely to be affected by this issue because of Medicare's policies governing enrollment in such plans. On the other hand, Medicare HMO enrollees in our sample appeared to be relatively satisfied with their coverage at the time of the survey, and empirically they were significantly less likely to enroll in TSSD.

The issue of Medigap reinstatement was highlighted in both our focus groups and in comments made by survey respondents. Focus group participants reported confusion about the conditions under which beneficiaries could reenroll in private Medigap programs at the conclusion of TSSD. Members of the RAND project team obtained information about the guidance given to program eligibles by staff members of the Iowa Foundation for Medical Care, who conducted informational meetings about the demonstration program in California and Texas. This information indicated that Medigap reinstatement rights were outlined in Section 4031 on Medigap Protections in the 1997 BBA. However, language in Section 722 of the fiscal year (FY) 1999 Defense Authorization Act lacks an explicit link between TSSD and any of the provisions in the 1997 BBA. This is in contrast to the language authorizing the FEHBP demonstration (Section 721 of the same legislation), which specifically states that enrollment in the FEHBP demonstration should be treated in the same way as enrollment in Medicare+Choice plans with respect to Medigap protections. To the extent that the BBA provisions do apply to TSSD, beneficiaries would have been entitled to return to Medigap plans A, B, C, or F, none of which cover prescription drugs, or to the beneficiary's last Medigap policy.

For reasons we described earlier, TSSD enrollees may have been overly optimistic about their rights to reinstate Medigap coverage at the end of the demonstration, particularly with respect to Medigap plans that cover prescription drugs or other enhanced benefits such as skilled nursing care. The practical consequences of any misunderstanding by beneficiaries are likely to be minor due to the new TFL benefits because the TFL program essentially eliminates the need for and value of private Medigap insurance. However, the confusion expressed by beneficiaries underscores the importance of providing accurate and comprehensive information about the full range of potential implications for beneficiaries who participate in DoD-sponsored demonstration programs, especially in light of the mistrust of the government expressed by many focus group participants and survey respondents.

Suitability of TSSD as a Permanent Program

When Congress instituted TFL, it deviated in many ways from the TSSD design. In addition to increasing the generosity of the health insurance benefit, Congress also altered the way it was administered. In particular, as with other private and employer-sponsored Medigap plans, coordination of claims between Medicare and TFL is automatic and does not require beneficiaries to file claims or deal with balance-billing.

In our view, the TFL model has substantial advantages for beneficiaries, relative to the TSSD model, in the the way that it is designed, and these advantages are unlikely to present major drawbacks for Medicare or the DoD. On the other hand, TSSD included some cost-sharing requirements, whereas TFL almost entirely eliminates cost-sharing for Medicare-covered services. Modest cost-sharing is likely to reduce health care use and thus the costs to the DoD of the benefit. At the same time, there is little definitive evidence that modest cost-sharing requirements are likely to have substantial negative effects on beneficiaries' health status. TSSD also included financial incentives to beneficiaries to use TRICARE network providers. Such a preferred-provider design provides some opportunities to manage care to improve efficiency, at least in principle (given the outcomes of TSSD, we could not assess this empirically).

Other Relevant Issues

The introduction of TFL significantly altered the policy context in which TSSD was being conducted, and with it our evaluation. We, therefore, focused on additional findings that may be relevant in the context of TFL.

- One key issue for TSSD, TFL, and other similar programs is the necessity for adequate decision support for beneficiaries. In TSSD—a demonstration program being conducted in two relatively confined geographic areas and with a clearly defined population of eligible beneficiaries—the DoD encountered difficulties in educating eligible beneficiaries about the demonstration. We found that a substantial fraction of nonenrolled beneficiaries claimed not to have heard of the demonstration, despite the efforts of the DoD and its contractors to inform beneficiaries about the program. In addition, lack of information was identified as one of the most important factors inhibiting TSSD participation among nonenrollees.

- A second issue, which we identified from our enrollment models, is the extent to which beneficiaries are likely to substitute DoD insurance benefits for existing supplemental coverage. Beneficiaries with existing employer-sponsored coverage were particularly unlikely to enroll in TSSD, whereas beneficiaries who had previously been purchasing private Medigap were relatively likely to enroll. This is consistent with our expectations regarding the relative value to beneficiaries of the various insurance options. In general, TFL has both more-generous benefits and lower out-of-pocket costs than TSSD, and more important, more-generous benefits and lower out-of-pocket costs than any private Medigap plan, employer-sponsored supplement, or Medicare HMO. As a result, it seems likely that beneficiaries with any of these plans, including employer-sponsored coverage, will drop such coverage in favor of TFL.

Conclusions

Given the existence of TFL and the accompanying pharmacy benefit program, the TRICARE Senior Supplement Demonstration is very unlikely to be implemented on a permanent national basis. However, in our view, the TSSD benefit design does present a viable model for a permanent national program for providing supplemental health insurance benefits to Medicare-eligible military retirees.

Advantages of TSSD

The TSSD benefits were comprehensive, the costs to beneficiaries were relatively low compared with most privately purchased Medigap plans and were comparable with many employer-sponsored supplemental policies, and the program could be administered on a national basis (unlike some of the other demonstration models for this population, particularly TRICARE Senior Prime and the Uniformed Services Family Health Plan). In addition, the modest cost-sharing requirements and the preferred-provider benefit design were consistent with many employer-sponsored supplemental policies, and unlike TFL in general, created some opportunities to further manage care and control program costs.

Areas for Improvement

Some features of the TRICARE Senior Supplement design could be improved:

- One improvement would be to institute automatic claims processing between Medicare and TSSD, as is done with other Medigap and supplemental policies (and TFL). The current procedures not only deterred enrollment and frustrated enrollees, they were so difficult for the DoD to implement that TMA stopped marketing TSSD in the summer of 2000.
- A second improvement would be to make the out-of-pocket costs associated with the use of nonnetwork providers more transparent to beneficiaries. This issue becomes less important the larger the TRICARE network is, and a permanent national TRICARE Senior Supplement program might induce additional providers to join the TRICARE network.

Low Awareness Among Beneficiaries

More generally, the findings from our evaluation highlight the difficulty of disseminating information about new, and complex, benefit programs. Despite efforts to publicize the program, awareness of TSSD seems to have been low among eligible beneficiaries, and understanding of the benefit design was imperfect even among enrollees.

Drawbacks Associated with a Temporary Demonstration

Finally, the findings illustrate the difficulties associated with accurately assessing demand for a health insurance program through a temporary demonstration. Many beneficiaries who were eligible for TSSD appeared to be reluctant to switch plans because they were familiar with their current plan and in many cases were very satisfied with it. TSSD may not have been sufficiently attractive as a temporary benefit to warrant the costs of switching insurance and then having to switch again at the end of the demonstration.

Beneficiaries were also reluctant to risk the possibility that their post-demonstration benefits would be worse than the status quo, and indeed there was ambiguity about whether TSSD enrollees would have a statutory right to return to their prior Medigap insurance after the demonstration. The impending availability of TFL should have reduced this concern (although TFL was not well understood at the time of our survey), but it may also have made beneficiaries more willing to retain their current coverage until TFL was available, rather than switching twice.

Future demonstration programs for this population would benefit from having these issues addressed as clearly and comprehensively as possible.

A. Focus Group Recruitment Letters

As we noted in Chapter 3, we conducted focus groups with TSSD enrollees and nonenrolled eligible beneficiaries to collect information about their attitudes toward the demonstration, their reasons for enrolling or remaining unenrolled, and information on other factors related to their enrollment.

Potential focus group participants received a recruitment letter from RAND, followed by a phone call from RAND to confirm focus group participation. Samples of the recruitment letters sent to enrollees and nonenrollees appear on the following pages.

Recruitment Letter for TSSD Enrollees

Dear <<TSSD participant>>:

You are invited to participate in a focus group discussion of the TRICARE Senior Supplement, your Military Health System benefits, and your health insurance needs.

As you may know, the Department of Defense is currently conducting the TRICARE Senior Supplement Demonstration program in your area. This program permits Military Health System beneficiaries who are receiving Medicare to enroll in TRICARE as a supplement to Medicare. This focus group is part of a study, sponsored by the Department of Defense, aimed at helping the federal government better understand the implementation of this program.

The Department of Defense has asked RAND to conduct this study. RAND is an independent, non-profit research organization with a national reputation for quality health care research.

The focus group, to be held on <DATE>, will include program participants and RAND researchers. During this meeting, you will have the opportunity to share your experiences with and thoughts about TRICARE Senior Supplement, your Military Health System benefits, and your health insurance needs, in a casual environment and with complete confidentiality. *As a participant in the TRICARE demonstration program, your views and experiences are extremely valuable in helping the Department of Defense and Congress improve health insurance benefits for military retirees and their families. Your input will greatly help the Military Health System to better serve military retirees and their families.*

The focus group will be held on <DATE> from <TIME1> until <TIME2> at <PLACE>. (Continental breakfast/Lunch) will be provided. To compensate you for your time, all attendees will receive $40.

You were randomly selected from a list of program participants. Although we hope you will join us, participation is voluntary. If you choose not to attend, it will not affect the benefits that you and your family receive, including your eligibility for the TRICARE demonstration program. Please be assured that anything you say during the focus group will be kept strictly confidential, and that RAND will not release any information that can be linked to you.

A member of the RAND research team will be contacting you by telephone to give you more details about this important event and answer any questions you may have about the study. You are also welcome to call us toll free at <1-800-XXX-XXXX>.

We hope that you will be able to join us for this important discussion.

Recruitment Letter for Nonenrolled TSSD Eligible Beneficiaries

Dear <<TSSD eligible>>:

You are invited to participate in a focus group discussion of TRICARE Senior Supplement, your Military Health System benefits, and your health insurance needs.

As you may know, the Department of Defense is currently conducting the TRICARE Senior Supplement Demonstration program in your area. This program permits Military Health System beneficiaries who are receiving Medicare to enroll in TRICARE as a supplement to Medicare.

This focus group is part of a study, sponsored by the Department of Defense, aimed at helping the federal government better understand the implementation of this program.

The Department of Defense has asked RAND to conduct this study. RAND is an independent, non-profit research organization with a national reputation for quality health care research.

The focus group, to be held on <DATE>, will include eligible beneficiaries and RAND researchers. During this meeting, you will have the opportunity to share your experiences with and thoughts about TRICARE Senior Supplement, your Military Health System benefits, and your health insurance needs, in a casual environment and with complete confidentiality. *Your views and experiences are extremely valuable in helping the Department of Defense and Congress improve health insurance benefits for military retirees and their families. Your input will greatly help the Military Health System to better serve military retirees and their families.*

The focus group will be held on <DATE> from <TIME1> until <TIME2> at <PLACE>. (Continental breakfast/Lunch) will be provided. To compensate you for your time, all attendees will receive $40.

You were randomly selected from a list of eligible beneficiaries. Although we hope you will join us, participation is voluntary. If you choose not to attend, it will not affect the benefits that you and your family receive, including your eligibility for the TRICARE demonstration program. Please be assured that anything you say during the focus group will be kept strictly confidential, and that RAND will not release any information that can be linked to you.

A member of the RAND research team will be contacting you by telephone to give you more details about this important event and answer any questions you may have about the study. You are also welcome to call us toll free at <1-800-XXX-XXXX>.

We hope that you will be able to join us for this important discussion.

B. Mail Survey Cover Letters and Sponsor Endorsement Letter

The evaluation activities for this study included a mail survey of TSSD enrollees and eligible nonenrolled beneficiaries. This appendix contains samples of the covering letters for the mail survey questionnaires that were sent to focus group attendees and beneficiaries who did not participate in the focus group and a sample of the accompanying sponsor endorsement letter.

Letter to Focus Group Attendees

DATE

FNAME LNAME

ADDRESS

Dear TITLE LNAME:

Recently we contacted you to invite you to attend a focus group discussion on military health benefits and the TRICARE Senior Supplement Demonstration Program. *We are now writing to ask for your help again!*

As you may recall, RAND, an independent non-profit research organization, is conducting a study on behalf of the Department of Defense regarding the health care benefits available to military retirees and their families. As before, you have been selected from a list obtained from the Department of Defense of military retirees who are either eligible to participate or who are enrolled in the TRICARE Senior Supplement Demonstration Program. The program, which is currently being implemented in your area, permits military retirees who are receiving Medicare to enroll in TRICARE as a supplement to Medicare. This study is aimed at helping the Department of Defense better understand how to successfully implement this program.

Enclosed you will find a questionnaire. We ask that you complete and return it in the postage-paid envelope as soon as possible. Even if you completed a similar questionnaire during the focus group, we ask that you do so again since this questionnaire contains new items.

As a military retiree who is eligible to receive health care benefits from the military, your experiences with and views regarding your health care coverage are extremely valuable to the Department of Defense and Congress as they work on improving the health care benefits offered to military retirees and their families.

While your input is invaluable, your participation in this study is voluntary. If you choose not to participate, it will not affect the benefits that you and your family personally receive, including your eligibility for the TRICARE Senior Supplement Demonstration Program. **Please be assured that RAND will keep your responses strictly confidential, and that RAND will not release any information that can be linked to you.**

If you have any questions about the study or have trouble completing the questionnaire, please call XXX toll free at 1-800-XXX-XXXX.

We look forward to your input on this very important issue.

Sincerely,

Letter to Beneficiaries Who Did Not Attend the Focus Groups

DATE

FNAME LNAME

ADDRESS

Dear TITLE LNAME:

We are writing to ask you to participate in a timely study regarding the health care benefits available to military retirees and their families. RAND, an independent non-profit research organization with a national reputation for quality health care research, is conducting this study on behalf of the Department of Defense.

You were selected to participate in this study from a list obtained from the Department of Defense of military retirees who are either eligible to participate or who are enrolled in the TRICARE Senior Supplement Demonstration Program. As you may know, the Department of Defense is currently implementing this program in your area. The program permits military retirees who are receiving Medicare to enroll in TRICARE as a supplement to Medicare. This study is aimed at helping the Department of Defense better understand how to successfully implement this program.

Enclosed you will find a questionnaire. We ask that you complete and return it in the postage paid envelope as soon as possible.

As a military retiree who is eligible to receive health care benefits from the military, your experiences with and views regarding your health care coverage are extremely valuable to the Department of Defense and Congress as they work on improving the health care benefits offered to military retirees and their families.

While your input is invaluable, your participation in this study is voluntary. If you choose not to participate, it will not affect the benefits that you and your family personally receive, including your eligibility for the TRICARE Senior Supplement Demonstration Program. **Please be assured that RAND will keep your responses strictly confidential, and that RAND will not release any information that can be linked to you.**

If you have any questions about the study or have trouble completing the questionnaire, please call XXXX toll free at 1-800-XXX-XXXX.

We look forward to your input on this very important issue.

Sincerely,

Sponsor Endorsement Letter

DATE

Dear <Beneficiary>:

The Department of Defense is currently conducting the TRICARE Senior Supplement Demonstration program in your area. This program permits Military Health System beneficiaries who are receiving Medicare to enroll in TRICARE as a supplement to Medicare. We have asked RAND, an independent non-profit research organization based in Santa Monica, California, to evaluate the success of this program. To do this, RAND researchers will be collecting information directly from program participants and other eligible beneficiaries, to hear their thoughts about the benefits and drawbacks of the program.

I am writing to you today to strongly encourage you to participate in RAND's evaluation efforts. *Why is it important for you to participate? Because your opinions matter!* Learning about your health insurance needs and your experiences with the Military Health System will help the Department of Defense and Congress improve benefits for military retirees and their families.

I want to emphasize that your participation in this evaluation is voluntary and will not affect the benefits that you and your family receive. Please be assured that all information collected from you will be kept strictly confidential, and that RAND will not release any information that can be linked to you.

Thank you in advance for your participation in this very important effort!

Sincerely,

<<project sponsor>>

C. Focus Group Protocol

As part of the focus group protocol for this study, each focus group session began with introductions and a description of the purpose of the TSSD pilot test. Confidentiality issues were discussed and participants were reminded of the voluntary nature of their participation. Participants were instructed to flag any questions that were unclear or difficult to answer and write their comments in the margin of the questionnaire. Participants were asked to spend up to 30 minutes on the questionnaire. The complete focus group protocol, which follows, was approved by RAND's Human Subjects Protection Committee.

Note: Text in the protocol that pertains to nonenrollees appears in italics.

Good morning. I am X, the moderator of today's focus group. Thank you for coming. I am with RAND in Washington, D.C. RAND is a non-profit research institution. I also have XX here with me today and she will be participating in our discussion.

<We would like to talk about your experiences so far in the TRICARE Senior Supplement Program./ *We would like to talk to you today about your health insurance coverage.*> This discussion is part of a larger study of the TRICARE Senior Supplement Program undertaken by RAND on behalf of the Department of Defense. The Department of Defense is seeking to better understand how to improve health care services to military retirees like yourselves.

Before we begin the discussion, I would like to take the first 15 or 20 minutes to have you fill out a questionnaire that we plan to administer to military retirees like yourselves who live in your area. Filling out this questionnaire will help you to start thinking about the issues we are here to discuss and will help us to identify and fix any questions that are difficult to answer before distributing the questionnaire more broadly.

The responses you provide in the questionnaire as well as your comments during the discussion that will follow are confidential—we won't be associating your names with what you say here. Please do not write your name on the questionnaire. Also, during our discussion today I would like everyone to use first names only. Because this discussion is confidential, I ask that during our discussion you not use specific names of individuals, and this includes your doctor, administrators of your health plan, or any other person. When the discussion is over, please respect the privacy of your fellow group members and do not repeat comments others make during our discussion to anyone outside of this group.

We are taping this discussion today so we don't have to take detailed notes. Does anyone have any objection to this taping?

Only people working on this project will ever hear any of the recordings, read the notes we take or have access to the questionnaire you complete. Your participation is voluntary and confidential, and you may refuse to comment on any question that is asked. Nothing you say about yourself, a particular person, or facility will ever be made public or reported in any way that will allow you to be identified. Your participation today will not affect the care that you and your family receive. So feel free to say whatever is on your mind.

Before we begin I want to emphasize that you are the experts here today. The reason we are here today is to better understand your experiences in <the TRICARE Senior Supplement Program/*with your health insurance coverage*>. There are no right or wrong answers. We want to hear what you think. During the discussion, I'm not planning on doing most of the talking. I do want to make sure that we cover a number of topics in a limited amount of time, so I'll try to keep things moving. There is no need to raise hands. Speak right up. But please respect others when they are talking.

Our time together may last up to about 90 minutes. Is there anyone who can't stay? Before we begin, are there any questions about how we will be conducting this discussion?

We'll start with the questionnaire.

1. Please answer all of the questions as best you can. Some questions ask you about past events and others refer to your spouse; your best guess in answering these questions is fine.

2. Please mark any questions that you do not understand/or are hard for you to answer with one of the sticky pieces of yellow paper (show an example).

3. If you finish early, please feel free to get up and walk around to stretch your legs or get a snack, but please refrain from talking so others may finish.

4. Don't worry if you haven't finished after 20 minutes, you are welcome to stay after the discussion and answer the remaining questions, but you don't have to.

5. Once you have completed the questionnaire, please hold on to it because we will refer to it in the discussion. However, please do not go back and change any of your answers. We will collect the questionnaires at the end of the discussion.

Now let's begin our discussion.

For enrollees: Today's discussion is part of our research into some details of the TRICARE Senior Supplement Program. As all of you probably know, the TRICARE Senior Supplement Program is a health insurance option offered by the Department of Defense to military retirees and retired spouses who are also eligible for Medicare. It is currently available in two areas of the country, including where you live. The plan is like a private Medigap supplement that covers prescription drugs.

I want to reiterate to you that we do not represent TRICARE or any of its programs. If you have any specific concerns or issues you need to discuss with a TRICARE representative, at the end of the discussion we can give you a toll-free number where you can reach a TRICARE representative.

For nonenrollees: Today's discussion is part of our research into some details of the TRICARE Senior Supplement Program. I understand that you are not enrolled in this plan; we are conducting other discussions with people who are. For those of you who may not know, the TRICARE Senior Supplement Program is a health insurance option offered by the Department of Defense to military retirees and retired spouses who are also eligible for Medicare. It is currently available in two areas of the country, including where you live. The plan is like a private Medigap supplement that covers prescription drugs.

I want to reiterate to you that we do not represent TRICARE or any of its programs. However, if you are interested in finding out more about the TRICARE Senior Supplement Program, please see one of us after the discussion and we will give you a toll-free number or Web site address where you can get more information.

1. Let's start by going around the room and introducing yourself. Please tell us two things about yourself: (1) your first name, and (2) how long you have been enrolled in the <TRICARE/*your current health insurance coverage*>.

2. What type of health insurance coverage did you have before enrolling in <the TRICARE Senior Supplement Program/*your current plan*>?

3. Please turn to page X in the questionnaire. This page contains a list of many of the features that people consider important in choosing a health plan. We have written the same list on this flip chart. How important were these

factors in your decision to enroll in <the TRICARE Senior Supplement Program/*your current plan*>?

How many people picked X as most important?

How many people picked X as least important?

Probe for trade-offs, i.e., I noticed that many people say that low premiums and drug coverage are very important. However, it is rare that health plans offer both. If you can't have both, which would you choose? Why?

> Note: options include:

> > Low monthly premiums

> > Coverage for care outside the United States

> > Low out-of-pocket costs for doctor office visits

> > Low out-of-pocket costs for hospital stays

> > Coverage of preventive services

> > Being able to choose my physician

> > Being able to choose my hospital

> > Coverage for mental health services

> > Spending a minimum amount of time on paperwork

> > Coverage for prescription drugs

4. How satisfied have you been so far with <the TRICARE Senior Supplement Program/*your current plan*>?

   What are the plusses? minuses?

   How does this compare to other plans you have been enrolled in?

5. In your opinion, why don't more military retirees like yourselves enroll in TSSD?

6. Questions related to Defense Appropriations Bill (NOTE: The Bill is not mentioned specifically):

   a. How would the availability of a low-cost prescription drug benefit through the military health care system affect your interest, or that of people like you, in the TRICARE Senior Supplement Program?

   b. How would the availability of a fee-for-service Medigap plan through the military health care system affect your interest, or that of people like you, in the TRICARE Senior Supplement Program?

   c. How would the availability of increased access to care at <CLOSEST MTF> affect your interest, or that of people like you, in the TRICARE Senior Supplement Program?

Finally, is there anything I haven't asked you that I should have?

Thank you very much for helping us out today. Your feedback will be very useful to us as we try to help the Department of Defense understand the health care needs of military retirees. It is all right to talk to others about what we discussed here today, but please remember to respect each other's privacy, and don't mention anyone's name outside this room.

If we have any additional questions or need clarification on any the points that were made today, may we contact you?

Would you like to receive a copy of the final report?

If you would like more information about the study, or if you would like to discuss any of these issues further, please don't hesitate to contact us at RAND: (800) xxx-xxxx. If you have time, we would be grateful if you would stay an extra couple of minutes to discuss the items in the questionnaire that you had difficulty answering. Otherwise, you are free to go.

D. Medigap Continuation Language from the TSSD Handbook

This appendix documents information, provided to TSSD eligible beneficiaries, that appears on the TRICARE Web site with regard to Medigap continuation. Concerns about program eligibles' perceptions about the guarantees of Medigap continuation are discussed in Chapter 6.

Current Language

The following text is current language from a publication titled *The TRICARE Senior Supplement Demonstration Program: Extending Your Health Care Benefits.* The publication is on the TSSD Web site at http://www.tricare.osd.mil/tssd/ (click "TRICARE Senior Supplement Handbook").

Will I need to maintain a supplemental or Medigap insurance?

That decision is personal, and should be based on a number of factors including your current health. Please remember that this is a demonstration program that is currently scheduled to end on December 31, 2002.

There are certain, limited situations where there would be protection in terms of reinstatement with a Medigap policy. Carriers differ in their policies with respect to your Medigap and supplemental policy reinstatement rights. Please check with your current carrier for specific information on your reinstatement rights.

Earlier Language

The following text appeared in an earlier version of *The TRICARE Senior Supplement Demonstration Program* document on the TSSD Web site.

Will I need to maintain a supplemental or Medigap insurance?

That decision is personal, and should be based on a number of factors including your current health. Please remember that this is a demonstration program that is currently scheduled to end on December 31, 2002. There are certain, limited situations where there would be protection in terms of reinstatement with a Medigap policy. What follows is from the Balanced Budget Act of 1997:

Guarantee Issuance: If an individual described below seeks to enroll in a Medigap policy within 63 days of the events described below, the issuer may not (1) deny or condition the issuance of a Medigap policy that is offered or available, (2) discriminate in the pricing of such a policy because of health status, claims experience, receipt of health care, or medical condition, and (3) impose a preexisting condition exclusion.

Guarantees issuance of Medigap plans "A," "B," "C," "F" or the Medicare supplemental policy that the individual was most recently previously enrolled in, if the individual: (1) was enrolled under a Medigap policy; (2) subsequently terminates such enrollment and enrolls with a Medicare+Choice organization, a risk or cost contract HMO, a similar organization operating under a demonstration project authority or a Medicare SELECT policy; and (3) terminates the Medicare+Choice enrollment within 12 months, but only if the individual was never previously enrolled with a Medicare+Choice entity.

Guarantees issuance of any Medigap plan to an individual who upon first becoming eligible for Medicare at age 65, enrolled in a Medicare+ Choice plan, and disenrolled from such plan within 12 months of the effective date of such enrollment.

E. Sample TSSD Mail Survey Instrument

This appendix reproduces the actual survey sent to TSSD enrollees and eligible nonenrolled beneficiaries as part of our evaluation of the TRICARE Senior Supplement Demonstration. The survey was prepared by RAND's Center for Military Health Policy Research.

Note: The following survey instrument was sent to individuals in the Santa Clara County, California, TSSD demonstration site. The survey used for the Cherokee County, Texas, demonstration site was the same as the California survey except that it omitted questions regarding Medicare+Choice HMO plans.

INSTRUCTIONS

About This Questionnaire

The information being collected in this questionnaire will help the Department of Defense better serve the healthcare needs of military retirees and their families. The responses you provide in this questionnaire are confidential. RAND will not release any of the information you report in such a way that it could be linked to you. **Please do not write your name on the questionnaire.**

Completing This Questionnaire

Please answer all of the questions as best you can. Some questions ask you about past events and others refer to your spouse. Your best guess in answering these questions is fine. At the beginning of each section, you will find a written introduction with additional instructions of how to complete that particular section. Please read these instructions carefully.

☞ You will also find instructions on how to complete a particular question immediately following that question. These instructions appear in *italics*.

☞ Most of the questions are followed by a list of responses from which you are asked to choose your answer by placing an ✗ or ✓ in the ❑ corresponding to your choice.

☞ If your response is other than those specifically listed, you are asked to include more information in the line provided as follows:
❑ Other *(please specify)*: _____

☞ For a few other questions, you are asked to write your answer in a ☐ .

☞ For some questions, responses are immediately followed by specific instructions in ***italics*** on whether to go to the next question or to skip to another question or page.

Questions or Comments

If you have any questions or comments regarding this questionnaire, please call Ana Suarez at RAND toll free at 800-255-6935. You can also provide written comments next to a specific question or on the last page of the questionnaire.

Returning the Questionnaire

Please return your completed questionnaire to RAND in the self-addressed and stamped envelope included with this questionnaire. If you do not have this envelope, please call us toll free at 800-255-6935 and we will send you another one.

PLEASE TURN TO PAGE 1

Section A:
Your Use of Health Care Services

This first set of questions is about your use of medical care.   Please tell us about your use of health care services, not that of your spouse or any other family member.

A1. **In the past YEAR, about how many times, if any, did <u>you</u> stay overnight for one or more nights in a hospital?**

> *(Check One)*
>
> ₁☐ None
>
> ₂☐ 1 time
>
> ₃☐ 2 to 4 times
>
> ₄☐ 5 or more times
>
> ₅☐ Don't know

A2. **In the past YEAR, about how many times did <u>you</u> visit an emergency room for medical care?**

> *(Check One)*
>
> ₁☐ None
>
> ₂☐ 1 time
>
> ₃☐ 2 to 4 times
>
> ₄☐ 5 or more times
>
> ₅☐ Don't know

A3. **In the past YEAR, about how many times did <u>you</u> visit a doctor or other medical professional in an office or clinic?** *Please do not include visits to the emergency room, hospital or dentist, or visits for eyeglasses or contact lenses.*

> *(Check One)*
>
> ₁☐ None
>
> ₂☐ 1 time
>
> ₃☐ 2 to 4 times
>
> ₄☐ 5 to 9 times
>
> ₅☐ 10 or more times
>
> ₆☐ Don't know

100

A4. How many prescription drugs are <u>you</u> currently taking?

(Check One)

- ₁❑ None
- ₂❑ 1 to 2 prescriptions
- ₃❑ 3 to 4 prescriptions
- ₄❑ 5 or more prescriptions
- ₅❑ Don't know

A5. In the past YEAR, where did you fill or refill most of <u>your</u> prescriptions?

(Check All That Apply)

- ₁❑ Military pharmacy
- ₂❑ Military mail-order program
- ₃❑ Civilian pharmacy or mail-order program
- ₄❑ VA pharmacy or mail-order program
- ₅❑ Other *(please specify)*: _____
- ₆❑ Don't know

A6. Over the past 5 YEARS, about how much of <u>your own</u> health care was at military health care facilities (excluding visits to the pharmacy)? *Please do NOT include care at VA facilities.*

(Check One)

- ₁❑ None
- ₂❑ Some
- ₃❑ Most
- ₄❑ All
- ₅❑ Don't know

Section B:

Health Plan Features and Benefits You Prefer

B1. **Choosing a health care insurance plan can be difficult. Desirable plans are often very expensive. How important are the following features to you in choosing a health plan?** *You may find it helpful to read through the entire list of features before answering.*

(Check One Box For Each Statement)

	Don't Need	Desirable But Not Necessary	Must Have
a. Low monthly premiums	₁ ☐	₂ ☐	₃ ☐
b. Coverage for care outside of the U.S.	₁ ☐	₂ ☐	₃ ☐
c. Low out-of-pocket costs for doctor office visits....	₁ ☐	₂ ☐	₃ ☐
d. Low out-of-pocket costs for hospital stays.............	₁ ☐	₂ ☐	₃ ☐
e. Coverage of preventive services	₁ ☐	₂ ☐	₃ ☐
f. Being able to choose my physician.......................	₁ ☐	₂ ☐	₃ ☐
g. Being able to choose my hospital..........................	₁ ☐	₂ ☐	₃ ☐
h. Coverage for mental health services	₁ ☐	₂ ☐	₃ ☐
i. Spending little or no time on paperwork	₁ ☐	₂ ☐	₃ ☐
j. Low out-of-pocket costs for prescription drugs	₁ ☐	₂ ☐	₃ ☐
k. Being able to keep my current physician(s)	₁ ☐	₂ ☐	₃ ☐

B2. **Please refer back to your responses to Question B1 above. Of the features that you "must have", which <u>two</u> are the most important to you?** *Please enter the <u>letters</u> that correspond to the two most important ones. Please enter only one <u>letter</u> in each box.*

Your response → The <u>two most</u> important to me are ☐ and ☐

B3. **Again, please refer back to your responses to Question B1 above. Of the features that you find "desirable but not necessary" or that you "don't need", which <u>two</u> are the least important to you?** *Please enter only one <u>letter</u> in each box.*

Your response → The <u>two least</u> important to me are ☐ and ☐

B4. How strongly do you agree or disagree with the following statements?

(Check One Box For Each Statement)

	Strongly Agree	Agree	Neither Agree Nor Disagree	Disagree	Strongly Disagree	Can't Say
a. Military retirees and their dependents can count on getting care at military treatment facilities when they need it.	1 ☐	2 ☐	3 ☐	4 ☐	5 ☐	6 ☐
b. Military retirees and their dependents age 65 and over should have the option of enrolling in TRICARE.................................	1 ☐	2 ☐	3 ☐	4 ☐	5 ☐	6 ☐
c. Military retirees and their dependents should contribute to the cost of their health care..................	1 ☐	2 ☐	3 ☐	4 ☐	5 ☐	6 ☐
d. Compared to other employers, the Military provides its retirees age 65 and over with generous health benefits....	1 ☐	2 ☐	3 ☐	4 ☐	5 ☐	6 ☐
e. Assuming that cost is not an issue, I prefer to have military-sponsored health care.	1 ☐	2 ☐	3 ☐	4 ☐	5 ☐	6 ☐

| Section C: |
| Your Health Insurance Coverage |

This section is about Medicare as well as any other health insurance coverage that <u>you</u> may have at this time, other than TRICARE sponsored plans.

C1. Are <u>you</u> currently covered by Medicare?

(Check One)

- ₁ ☐ Yes → *GO TO QUESTION C2*
- ₂ ☐ No → *SKIP TO PAGE 7, QUESTION D1*
- ₃ ☐ Don't know → *SKIP TO PAGE 7, QUESTION D1*

C2. Medicare Part B helps pay for doctors' services and outpatient hospital services for an additional monthly premium. Are <u>you</u> currently enrolled in Medicare Part B?

(Check One)

- ₁ ☐ Yes
- ₂ ☐ No
- ₃ ☐ Don't know

C3. Several Medicare HMOs are available in your area as alternatives to traditional Medicare. Are <u>you</u> currently enrolled in a Medicare HMO (e.g., Senior Secure, Health Net Seniority Plus, Secure Horizons Standard, Secure Horizons Basic, Kaiser Permanente Senior Advantage, or another Medicare HMO)?

(Check One)

- ₁ ☐ Yes
- ₂ ☐ No
- ₃ ☐ Don't know

C4. Aside from Medicare and a TRICARE sponsored plan, do <u>you</u> currently have any of the following types of health insurance plan(s)?

> *(Check All That Apply)*

> 1 ☐ Medigap or Medicare supplement insurance purchased from an insurance company or agent.
> *Please specify plan letter:* ☐
>
> 2 ☐ A plan sponsored by former civilian employer or union
> 3 ☐ Medicaid
> 4 ☐ Other *(please specify)*: _____
> 5 ☐ None ➔ *SKIP TO NEXT PAGE, QUESTION D1*
> 6 ☐ Don't know ➔ *SKIP TO NEXT PAGE, QUESTION D1*

C5. Do any of the plans that you selected in Question C4 above cover prescription drugs?

> *(Check One)*

> 1 ☐ Yes
> 2 ☐ No
> 3 ☐ Don't know

➤

Section D:
TRICARE Senior Supplement Demonstration Program

TRICARE Senior Supplement is a demonstration program that allows retired Uniformed Services personnel and their family members who are age 65 and over to enroll, for a limited period of time, in TRICARE Standard or TRICARE Extra as a supplement to their Medicare coverage.

D1. Before receiving this questionnaire, did you (or your spouse) know about the TRICARE Senior Supplement Demonstration Program?

(Check One)

₁ ☐ Yes → *GO TO QUESTION D2*

₂ ☐ No → *SKIP TO PAGE 12, QUESTION E1*

₃ ☐ Not sure → *SKIP TO PAGE 12, QUESTION E1*

D2. How did you (or your spouse) learn about the TRICARE Senior Supplement Demonstration Program?

(Check All That Apply)

₁ ☐ Read information that the military mailed

₂ ☐ Got information from an organization that represents military retirees or their families

₃ ☐ Heard about it from my Congressman's office

₄ ☐ Attended a health fair or town meeting

₅ ☐ Heard about the demonstration on radio or television

₆ ☐ Read an article about the demonstration in the local newspaper

₇ ☐ Heard about the demonstration from family or friends

₈ ☐ Other *(please specify)*: _____

₉ ☐ Not sure

D3. Did you (or your spouse) have trouble deciding whether or not to join the TRICARE Senior Supplement Demonstration Program?

(Check One)

₁ ☐ Yes → *GO TO QUESTION D4, NEXT PAGE*

₂ ☐ No → *SKIP TO QUESTION D5, NEXT PAGE*

₃ ☐ Not sure → *SKIP TO QUESTION D5, NEXT PAGE*

D4. Why did you (or your spouse) have trouble deciding whether or not to join the TRICARE Senior Supplement Demonstration Program?

(Check All That Apply)

₁❏ Wasn't sure how much the plan would really cost

₂❏ Couldn't tell how the plan would work with Medicare benefits

₃❏ It was hard to understand what services the plan covered

₄❏ It was hard to understand which physicians and hospitals were covered

₅❏ It was hard to tell how much paperwork is required

₆❏ It was hard to compare TRICARE Senior Supplement to other plans

₇❏ Concerned about dropping my (our) other insurance

₈❏ Other *(please specify)*: _____

₉❏ Can't say

D5. Are _you_ currently enrolled in the TRICARE Senior Supplement Demonstration Program?
Please answer this question about yourself, not your spouse.

(Check One)

₁❏ Yes ➔ *SKIP TO PAGE 10, QUESTION D8*

₂❏ No ➔ *GO TO QUESTION D6, NEXT PAGE*

₃❏ Don't know ➔ *SKIP TO PAGE 12, QUESTION E1*

For non-participants in the TRICARE Senior Supplement Demonstration Program

Answer the following questions if <u>you are not currently enrolled</u> in the TRICARE Senior Supplement Demonstration Program. If <u>you are currently enrolled</u> in the TRICARE Senior Supplement Demonstration Program, please skip to page 10, Question D8.

D6. Why didn't <u>you</u> join the TRICARE Senior Supplement Demonstration Program?
(Check All That Apply)

1 ☐ I'm not eligible

2 ☐ I'm satisfied with my current coverage

3 ☐ I plan to enroll but have not done so yet

4 ☐ I dislike military health care

5 ☐ I wanted/needed benefits that are not covered by TRICARE Senior Supplement

6 ☐ I don't like any of the doctors in the TRICARE Extra network

7 ☐ I don't like having to file claims for reimbursement

8 ☐ I have not received enough information about TRICARE Senior Supplement

9 ☐ I live in another part of the country during the year

10 ☐ The coverage is only available for a limited period of time

11 ☐ Other *(please explain)*: _____

12 ☐ Not sure ➔ *SKIP TO PAGE 12, QUESTION E1*

D7. Of the reasons you gave in question D6 above, what are the <u>two</u> main reasons <u>you</u> didn't join the TRICARE Senior Supplement Demonstration Program? *Please refer back to your responses to the question above and enter the numbers that correspond with the two main reasons why <u>you</u> didn't join TRICARE Senior Supplement. Please enter only one <u>number</u> in each box.*

Your response ➔ The <u>two</u> main reasons I didn't join are ☐ and ☐

NOW GO TO PAGE 12, SECTION E.

For participants in the TRICARE Senior Supplement Demonstration Program

---

Answer the following questions if <u>you are currently enrolled</u> in the TRICARE Senior Supplement Demonstration Program. If <u>you are not currently enrolled</u> in the TRICARE Senior Supplement Demonstration Program, please skip to page 12, Section E.

D8. **Why did <u>you</u> join the TRICARE Senior Supplement Demonstration Program?**
(Check All That Apply)

1 ☐ It costs less than my previous coverage (insurance or health plan)

2 ☐ It costs less than other coverage that I could buy

3 ☐ The plan's benefits package meets my needs

4 ☐ The plan's benefits package is better than other coverage I could get

5 ☐ It offers a wide choice of physicians and hospitals

6 ☐ It offers better drug coverage

7 ☐ The plan has a good reputation for quality of care

8 ☐ I don't want to use military health care facilities

9 ☐ My friends or relatives recommended that I join the plan

10 ☐ It is more convenient if my spouse and I are in the same plan

11 ☐ I prefer to have military sponsored health care

12 ☐ Other *(please specify)*: _____

13 ☐ Not sure ➔ *SKIP TO PAGE 11, QUESTION D10*

D9. **Of the reasons you gave in question D8 above, what are the <u>two</u> main reason <u>you</u> joined the TRICARE Senior Supplement Demonstration Program?** *Please refer back to your responses to the question above and enter the numbers that correspond with the two main reasons why <u>you</u> joined TRICARE Senior Supplement. Please enter only one <u>number</u> in each box.*

Your response ➔ The <u>two</u> main reasons I joined are ☐ and ☐

D10. Overall, how satisfied are <u>you</u> with the TRICARE Senior Supplement Demonstration Program?

(Check One)

₁ ☐ Very satisfied

₂ ☐ Satisfied

₃ ☐ Not satisfied

₄ ☐ Can't say

D11. Aside from traditional Medicare, what type of health insurance plan(s) did <u>you</u> have <u>before you</u> enrolled in TRICARE Senior Supplement Demonstration Program?

(Check All That Apply)

₁ ☐ Medigap or Medicare supplement insurance purchased from an insurance company or agent.

                      Please specify plan letter: ☐

₂ ☐ A Medicare HMO

₃ ☐ A plan sponsored by former civilian employer or union

₄ ☐ Medicaid

₅ ☐ Other *(please specify)*: _____

₆ ☐ None ➔ *SKIP TO NEXT PAGE, QUESTION E1*

₇ ☐ Don't know ➔ *SKIP TO NEXT PAGE, QUESTION E1*

D12. Did any of the plans that you selected in Question D11 above cover prescription drugs?

(Check One)

₁ ☐ Yes

₂ ☐ No

₃ ☐ Don't know

110

Section E:
Your Health Status

The following questions are about <u>your</u> overall health.

E1. **In general, compared to other people your age, would you say your health is:**
    (Check One)
    - ₁❑ Excellent
    - ₂❑ Very good
    - ₃❑ Good
    - ₄❑ Fair
    - ₅❑ Poor
    - ₆❑ Can't say

E2. **Compared to 6 MONTHS ago, how would you rate your health in general <u>now</u>?**
    (Check One)
    - ₁❑ Much better now than 6 months ago
    - ₂❑ Somewhat better now than 6 months ago
    - ₃❑ About the same
    - ₄❑ Somewhat worse now than 6 months ago
    - ₅❑ Much worse now than 6 months ago
    - ₆❑ Can't say

E3. **Do you <u>expect</u> your health to be better or worse 6 MONTHS from now?**
    (Check One)
    - ₁❑ Better than today
    - ₂❑ About the same as today
    - ₃❑ Worse than today
    - ₄❑ Can't say

E4. During the past YEAR, did <u>you</u> have a serious illness, chronic condition, injury or disability that required a lot of medical care?

(Check One)

₁ ☐ Yes
₂ ☐ No
₃ ☐ Don't know

E5. During the past MONTH, how much of the time has <u>your</u> health limited social activities like visiting with friends or relatives?

(Check One)

₁ ☐ None of the time
₂ ☐ Some of the time
₃ ☐ Most of the time
₄ ☐ All of the time
₅ ☐ Can't say

112

E6. Has a doctor or other medical professional ever told you that you had any of the following medical conditions?

(Check All That Apply)

1 ❑ Hardening of the arteries or arteriosclerosis

2 ❑ High blood pressure or hypertension

3 ❑ Heart attack or myocardial infarction

4 ❑ Coronary heart disease

5 ❑ Congestive heart failure

6 ❑ Stroke, brain hemorrhage or cerebrovascular accident

7 ❑ Skin cancer

8 ❑ Cancer, malignancy, or tumor other than skin cancer

9 ❑ Diabetes, high blood sugar or sugar in your urine

10 ❑ Rheumatoid arthritis

11 ❑ Fragile bones or osteoporosis

12 ❑ Parkinson's disease

13 ❑ Emphysema, asthma, or chronic obstructive pulmonary disease

14 ❑ Complete or partial paralysis

15 ❑ None of the above

16 ❑ Don't know

E7. Because of impairment or health problems, how often do you need the help of other people with your personal care needs, such as eating, bathing/dressing, or getting around the house?

(Check One)

1 ❑ None of the time

2 ❑ Some of the time

3 ❑ Most of the time

4 ❑ All of the time

5 ❑ Can't say

Section F:
Facts About You and Your Family

The information you provide in this section will be used to study how different groups of people use health care services and military health benefits. This information will NOT be used to identify you personally.

F1. Are <u>you</u> male or female?

(Check One)

₁☐ Male

₂☐ Female

F2. How old were <u>you</u> on your last birthday?   Age: ☐☐

F3. How many people live in your household?   Number of people: ☐☐

F4. Do you (or your spouse) belong to an organization that represents military retirees and their families?

(Check One)

₁☐ Yes

₂☐ No

₃☐ Don't know

F5. What was <u>your</u> rank at the time of retirement from the military? *If you are eligible for military health care because of your own as well as your spouse's military services, please give <u>your own</u> rank.*

(Check One)

₁☐ Officer

₂☐ Warrant officer

₃☐ Non-commissioned officer

₄☐ Enlisted

₅☐ Other *(please specify)*: _____

₆☐ Don't know

114

F6. What is <u>your</u> race?

(Check One)

- ₁◻ White
- ₂◻ Black or African-American
- ₃◻ American Indian or Alaska Native
- ₄◻ Asian
- ₅◻ Native Hawaiian or other Pacific Islander
- ₆◻ Other *(please specify)*: _____

F7. Are <u>you</u> Hispanic, Latino or of Spanish origin?

(Check One)

- ₁◻ Yes
- ₂◻ No

F8. What is the highest grade or level of school that <u>you</u> have <u>completed</u>?

(Check One)

- ₁◻ 8th grade or less
- ₂◻ Some high school, but did not graduate
- ₃◻ High school graduate or GED
- ₄◻ Some college or 2-year degree
- ₅◻ 4-year college degree
- ₆◻ More than 4-year college degree

F9. In 2000, what was <u>your family's</u> **TOTAL income BEFORE taxes?** *Please include income from ALL sources such as work; pensions; dividend; annuities; interest; Social Security benefits; SSI; alimony; rental income and any other money income received by you or members of your family who are 15 years or older and living with you. Your best guess is fine.*

(Check One)

₁ ☐ Less than $20,000

₂ ☐ $20,000 to $39,999

₃ ☐ $40,000 to $59,999

₄ ☐ $60,000 to $79,999

₅ ☐ $80,000 and over

₆ ☐ Don't know

F10. **Other than health insurance premiums, approximately how much do you spend out of your own pocket on health care services for you (and your spouse) each YEAR?** *Your best guess is fine. Think about the money you (and your spouse) spend on co-pays, deductibles, prescription drugs and services not covered by your insurance plan. <u>Please do not include health insurance premiums</u>.*

(Check One)

₁ ☐ $0 to $99 per year

₂ ☐ $100 to $499 per year

₃ ☐ $500 to $999 per year

₄ ☐ $1000 to $4999 per year

₅ ☐ $5000 or more per year

₆ ☐ Don't know

F11. **Which of the following best describes your <u>current</u> marital status?**

(Check One)

₁ ☐ Married ➔ *GO TO SECTION G, NEXT PAGE*

₂ ☐ Never married

₃ ☐ Separated   ▶ *SKIP TO END, PAGE 24*

₄ ☐ Divorced

₅ ☐ Widowed

California   17

116

Section G:
Your Spouse

The following questions are about your spouse. Please answer them to the best of your knowledge.

G1. Is _your spouse_ currently covered by Medicare?

(Check One)

₁❑ Yes ➔ *GO TO QUESTION G2*

₂❑ No ➔ *SKIP TO END, PAGE 24*

₃❑ Don't know ➔ *SKIP TO PAGE 19, QUESTION G5*

G2. Is _your spouse_ currently enrolled in Medicare Part B?

(Check One)

₁❑ Yes

₂❑ No

₃❑ Don't know

G3. Several Medicare HMOs are available in your area as alternatives to traditional Medicare. Is _your spouse_ currently enrolled in a Medicare HMO (e.g., Senior Secure, Health Net Seniority Plus, Secure Horizons Standard, Secure Horizons Basic, Kaiser Permanente Senior Advantage, or another Medicare HMO)?

(Check One)

₁❑ Yes

₂❑ No

₃❑ Don't know

G4. Aside from Medicare and a TRICARE sponsored plan, does _your spouse_ currently have any of the following types of health insurance plan(s)?

(Check All That Apply)

₁❑ Medigap or Medicare supplement insurance purchased from an insurance company or agent.

Please specify plan letter: ☐

₂❑ A plan sponsored by former civilian employer or union

₃❑ Medicaid

₄❑ Other *(please specify)*: _____

₅❑ None

₆❑ Don't know

California   18

G5. In the past YEAR, how many times, if any, did <u>your spouse</u> stay overnight for one or more nights in a hospital?

(Check One)

- $_1$☐ None
- $_2$☐ 1 time
- $_3$☐ 2 to 4 times
- $_4$☐ 5 or more times
- $_5$☐ Don't know

G6. In the past YEAR, about how many times did <u>your spouse</u> visit an emergency room for medical care?

(Check One)

- $_1$☐ None
- $_2$☐ 1 time
- $_3$☐ 2 to 4 times
- $_4$☐ 5 or more times
- $_5$☐ Don't know

G7. In the past YEAR, about how many times did <u>your spouse</u> visit a doctor or other medical professional in an office or clinic? *Please do not include visits to the emergency room, hospital or dentist, or visits for eyeglasses or contact lenses.*

(Check One)

- $_1$☐ None
- $_2$☐ 1 time
- $_3$☐ 2 to 4 times
- $_4$☐ 5 to 9 times
- $_5$☐ 10 or more times
- $_6$☐ Don't know

118

G8. How many prescription drugs is <u>your spouse</u> currently taking?

(Check One)

₁❑ None

₂❑ 1 to 2 prescriptions

₃❑ 3 to 4 prescriptions

₄❑ 5 or more prescriptions

₅❑ Don't know

G9. Over the past 5 YEARS, about how much of <u>your spouse's</u> health care was at military health care facilities (excluding visits to the pharmacy)? *Please do NOT include care at VA facilities.*

(Check One)

₁❑ None

₂❑ Some

₃❑ Most

₄❑ All

₅❑ Don't know

G10.In general, compared to other people his/her age, would you say that <u>your spouse's</u> health is:

(Check One)

₁❑ Excellent

₂❑ Very good

₃❑ Good

₄❑ Fair

₅❑ Poor

₆❑ Can't say

G11.Compared to 6 MONTHS ago, how would you rate <u>your spouse's</u> health in general <u>now</u>?

(Check One)

- ₁❑ Much better now than 6 months ago
- ₂❑ Somewhat better now than 6 months ago
- ₃❑ About the same
- ₄❑ Somewhat worse now than 6 months ago
- ₅❑ Much worse now than 6 months ago
- ₆❑ Can't say

G12.During the past YEAR, did <u>your spouse</u> have a serious illness, chronic condition, injury or disability that required a lot of medical care?

(Check One)

- ₁❑ Yes
- ₂❑ No
- ₃❑ Don't know

G13.Because of impairment or health problems, how often does <u>your spouse</u> need the help of other people with <u>his/her</u> personal care needs, such as eating, bathing/dressing, or getting around the house?

(Check One)

- ₁❑ None of the time
- ₂❑ Some of the time
- ₃❑ Most of the time
- ₄❑ All of the time
- ₅❑ Can't say

G14.Is <u>your spouse</u> currently enrolled in the TRICARE Senior Supplement Demonstration Program?

(Check One)

- ₁❑ Yes ➔ *GO TO QUESTION G15, NEXT PAGE*
- ₂❑ No ➔ *SKIP TO PAGE 23, QUESTION G17*
- ₃❑ Don't know ➔ *SKIP TO END, PAGE 24*

120

G15. Why did <u>your spouse</u> join the TRICARE Senior Supplement Demonstration Program?

(Check All That Apply)

- ₁ ❑ It cost less than my spouse's previous coverage (insurance or health plan)
- ₂ ❑ It costs less than other coverage my spouse could buy
- ₃ ❑ The plan's benefits package meets the needs of my spouse
- ₄ ❑ The plan's benefits package is better than other coverage my spouse could get
- ₅ ❑ My spouse needed better coverage for prescriptions
- ₆ ❑ My spouse did not want to use military health care facilities
- ₇ ❑ Friends or relatives recommended it to my spouse
- ₈ ❑ It is more convenient if my spouse and I are in the same plan
- ₉ ❑ My spouse prefers to have military sponsored health care
- ₁₀ ❑ Other *(please explain)*: _____
- ₁₁ ❑ Don't know

G16. Overall, how satisfied is <u>your spouse</u> with the TRICARE Senior Supplement Demonstration Program?

(Check One)

- ₁ ❑ Very satisfied
- ₂ ❑ Satisfied
- ₃ ❑ Not satisfied
- ₄ ❑ Don't know

NOW SKIP TO END, PAGE 24

G17.Why didn't <u>your spouse</u> join the TRICARE Senior Supplement Demonstration Program?
(Check All That Apply)

₁❑ My spouse is not eligible

₂❑ My spouse is satisfied with his/her current coverage

₃❑ My spouse plan's to enroll but have not done so yet

₄❑ My spouse dislikes military health care

₅❑ My spouse wanted/needed benefits that are not covered by TRICARE Senior Supplement

₆❑ My spouse doesn't like any of the doctors in the TRICARE Extra network

₇❑ My spouse doesn't like having to file claims for reimbursement

₈❑ Other *(please explain)*: _____

₉❑ Don't know

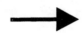

Is there anything else you would like to share with us? Your comments are greatly appreciated.

_____
_____
_____
_____
_____
_____
_____
_____
_____
_____
_____
_____
_____

Please return your completed survey to RAND in the self-addressed and stamped envelope provided. If you do not have this envelope, please call us toll-free at 800-255-6935 and we will send you another one.

It is not necessary for you to write your name and address on the envelope.

Please remember <u>not</u> to write your name anywhere on the questionnaire.

THANK YOU FOR YOUR PARTICIPATION IN THIS IMPORTANT STUDY!

F. Selected TSSD Survey Comments

In this appendix, we present a sampling of comments that we received from individuals who participated in the TSSD mail survey. We received comments from both TSSD enrollees and nonenrolled eligible beneficiaries who shared their opinions on several areas of the program.

Comments from Enrollees: Claims Processing

- So far, our claims have offered no benefits to providers or subscribers. To date, one claim going back to Nov. '00 has not been acknowledged (no explanation of benefits and no response to the provider). [Respondent appended an extract of similar thoughts expressed on another occasion.]

- There have been some problems [in] handling claims and a mix-up about my spouse's eligibility for coverage. It does appear, however, that some effort is being made to correct these problems.

- The payment to the provider is sometimes denied due to wrong codes, etc., and I can never get it straightened out. The paperwork becomes a nightmare and getting the payments straightened out is terrible. If you are not willing to spend hours [writing] letters you end up having to pay extra.

- I had numerous medical bills last year, but have yet to receive any payment from TSSD. The fact that I have another supplement may be part of the problem. A weak part of TSSD, I believe, is lack of benefit coordination with Medicare and/or other supplemental insurance.

- TRICARE Senior Supplement seems to be slow in paying physician[s].

- During the six months we were in TSSD, we submitted several small Medicare Supplement claims to PGBA [Palmetto Government Benefits Administrators, a fiscal intermediary for TRICARE] in Surfside Beach, S.C. Three were apparently lost, but just last week they paid one of them, six months afterwards. The fourth they apparently didn't recognize as a supplementary claim because they requested an itemized bill from the doctor. The fifth was actually processed, but since Medicare approved $83, and TRICARE allowed only $63 for that particular service, they didn't pay anything. This explains why we dropped out of TSSD.

- The TRICARE Senior Supplement Demo Program has paid NOTHING beyond what Medicare paid on any doctor's bill. Medicare pays 80% of its "Approved amt."; TRICARE does not pay this 20% difference or any part of the difference to the provider of services. The personnel responding to claim queries at Palmetto Government Benefit Administration are invariably polite but totally useless in resolving claim problems. Nor does anyone at the Information Systems of the Iowa Foundation for Medical Care seem able to answer fairly simple claim questions. All our TRICARE Explanation of Benefits Statements show: "Pd. To provider: 0, Pd. to beneficiary: 0, Check # _____."

- Claims took too long to process and payment to physicians was extremely long in coming.

- I learned that my doctor and I would have to prepare and submit the claim forms. Medicare would have automatically notified TRICARE after a procedure was completed, as [is] done with my current Medicare supplement carrier (USAA). I would reenroll in the TRICARE SSD program if some or all of these deficiencies were eliminated.

- TRICARE Senior Supplement should be tied to MEDICARE by computer and when Medicare pays the provider they (TRICARE) should make payment without further claim filing. If Medicare pays, TRICARE accepts their decision and pays the copay without paper work. During this demonstration, TRICARE Senior Supplement personnel were difficult to work with— demanding many unnecessary receipts when Medicare had already paid. It appears they were not knowledgeable of how Medicare works and that TRICARE Senior Supplement is "just that—a *supplement.*"

- [Respondent provided detailed history of efforts to have TSSD cover a particular claim that had been approved and paid by Medicare.] Observations: [Claims processor] is understaffed for this program. They pay nothing for at least 30 days. The persons answering inquiries know very little [about] how their system works or who to call in their company to correct mistakes. (A Medical Director would help.) It seems usual for the Medicare supplement insurer to deny payment after the primary insurer, Medicare, has paid. This situation never occurred in the many years we had private Medigap policies. There are no specific "Third-Party Forms" at any provider's office we have visited. We show the provider our insurance cards for their records. If the TRICARE-for-Life program begins in October 2001, it would be unfortunate if this load of claims processing was dumped on an already overworked system.

- From my 10-month experience with TRICARE SS Demonstration Program, I am thrilled with the performance of the Mail-In Pharmacy. They do an outstanding job in assisting and expediting. As a secondary payer, TRICARE now performs at the same satisfactory level that I previously enjoyed from BC/BS. TRICARE was a little shaky for the first X months particularly about paying reimbursement to plan members.

- The TSSD program was not prepared to handle the response load at the time it became available. The TSSD program had no provision for medical facilities to file *one* set of claim forms with Medicare and then be passed on to TRICARE for further processing. The TSSD still does not allow for direct bank draft[s] for payment of premiums.

- [Respondent listed recent medical history.] I listed all of this to emphasize what I consider a major problem with the TRICARE accounting. I have a huge stack of medical bills. I have received only a few statements from TRICARE paying minor amounts and refusing some! The way the charges are written it is almost impossible to tell what specific charges they are dealing with! It is a monumental task to identify what charges they have received and what info they should be sent for payment!

- My spouse and I both enrolled but disenrolled just prior to the start-up of TSSD. My spouse and I are preparing for, and looking forward to, TFL (TRICARE for Life), which we well deserve. Hopefully the program will include a provision for Medicare to pass on health care usage information to TRICARE, to *speed up payment* to providers and keep relationships good. TRICARE has a reputation of being slow payers. The best providers may require patients to pay up front and file their own TFL claim. Thank you for your help.

- Overall for me, we have been satisfied. But my wife (who has retirement insurance from her company) has *not* been happy with TRICARE. They simply do *not* pay. It takes several filings and then TRICARE may or may not choose to pay paltry amounts. Because of this, we've had more out-of-pocket [expenses] on my wife than we should [have]. TRICARE makes it too hard to receive payments for medical services. Thank goodness I'm very healthy!

- Having served as a warrant officer in the Marine Corps and being required to have an annual physical convinced me that annual physicals almost invariably discovered health problems in early stages. Since retiring from the Corps in 195X, my wife and I have had regular annual physicals. We are both in fairly good health. As to why we are dissatisfied with TSSD—I have a lousy small health insurance policy sponsored by a former civilian employer following retirement from military service. After enrolling in TSSD, every time we filed a claim or a pharmacist called TSSD for a prescription, the claim was flagged for [a] second payer. TSSD became [the] third payer and few if any doctors, pharmacists, or hospitals will file three claims. Our civilian health policy pays only in dire cases—usually for in-hospital cases. It was decided that I would be required to pay for prescriptions (full price), then get a list of our prescriptions from the pharmacy, signed by the registered pharmacist, make out a claim form, attach paid cash register receipts, mail them to [Medigap] (which does not pay on prescriptions), [Medigap] would reject the claim, then it would go to TSSD to pay. This placed all the burden of paying, doing all the paperwork, etc., on me. The concept of TSSD is great, and when it is made second payer after Medicare, I believe the above problem will be solved.

- Recommend that TRICARE establish a program with Medicare like TROA Mediplus. It requires no paperwork. After Medicare pays, it forwards paper (or online) to Mediplus who pays the required amount.

- Why can't it be set up so that Medicare will automatically file with TRICARE directly as it does with other Medigap policies? Would save a lot of time and confusion. Also, why won't TRICARE cover chiropractic care like Medicare and Medigaps [do]?

- My only problem has been that Medicare does not send the Medicare summary notices of what Medicare has paid on to TRICARE for supplementary payments—sometimes we have to bundle up all Medicare notices of payments along with paid receipts from [the] balance due the doctor to TRICARE for payment. This is time consuming. Medicare should be *required* to send this on to *TRICARE* so payment can be made automatically—the older we get, the more *paperwork* becomes a burden to us. TRICARE needs an *electronic* filing number. Our doctors say they can't file for us since TRICARE doesn't have an electronic number and they don't file any other way.

- Our dissatisfaction with this program arises with the EOB (the "E" is lacking). We find: (a) some terminology (copayment–coshare–TRICARE approved–deductible) is unclear or its use [is] confusing; (b) some "remarks" seem unclear or unnecessary, perhaps contradictory or even meaningless.

Comments from Enrollees: Cost/Coverage

- Previous insurance carrier was [affinity group supplement], which increased in cost from $150 a month in Feb. 2000, so [we] went to TSSD in May 2000 at a cost of $96 a month. FRA did cover all deductibles plus 20% that Medicare does not cover. Medicare notified FRA of all unpaid costs, which were then picked up and automatically paid. With TSSD, I am never sure if they will pay the 20% Medicare does not cover. I have sent in Medicare Summary notices. I have ended up paying the 20% rather than incur the wrath of billing offices and doctors. So far, from May 2000, I am out $1,152. TSSD so far has paid $131 and I have picked up an additional $72 (20% costs). There has to be a better way!!!!!

- Would like coverage for eyeglasses and hearing aids.

- COST: At age 65 they put us in Medicare A and B off CHAMPUS—charged us $49 or $100 [a month for] prescription coverage and TRSSO cost us $576 a year plus $8 for drugs for 3 months. Now, for free medical coverage think about this: $576 x 2 = $1,152 a year [and] $100 x 2 = $1,200 [for] Part B. $1,200 + $1,152 = $2,352 [that] I'm paying for free medical for lifetime?

- My only concern about the program is, as I travel and need medical help, will it be covered by [the] TRICARE Senior Supplement Program? One of my doctors refused to accept this program because of slow payments under the regular TRICARE program.

- The following should be provided [to] retired military families—dental care, hearing aids, glasses. Take some of [the] money going to [filthy rich] kings and dictators and fulfill promises made to military retirees!!!

- Since we have only been in the program about a year, and [have] no medical problems, we have very little to compare, except for the major savings on Medigap premiums and prescriptions—that will be a big help to us.

- This TSSD plan should cover eyeglasses, dental plan, [and] hearing aids as it is a Senior Citizen plan and all seniors need at least one of these items.

Comments from Enrollees: General

- I am very pleased with TSSD and pray that it continues. I have recommended the plan to my friends.

- We are very satisfied with TRICARE!!

- We appreciate the TRICARE Program. It is beneficial and most helpful to us since we are many miles away from any military hospital.

- We hope that the TRICARE program will be implemented nationally. We're pleased to have participated in the demonstration. We hope that the TRICARE program will become generally available to all eligible military retirees. Within the past few days, we were "disenrolled" from TSSD because we moved to a retirement home in the adjacent county. That turn of affairs was disappointing. We certainly will reenroll in TRICARE whenever it becomes possible.

- I think this is a great program. The national mail order pharmacy is a most important benefit to us.

- TRICARE Senior Supplement has been good.

- My wife and I are *very* pleased to have the opportunity to belong to the TRICARE Senior demonstration program. The prescription drug (mail order) has been especially helpful. THANKS!

- A long way from free but [it] is a good plan.

- 1. I still don't know how the $150 deductible is implemented! I think it should be same as Medicare. 2. Several doctors don't know about TRICARE SSD. They know or have heard about CHAMPUS. 3. I'm not sure what is the procedure for filing for drug reimbursement when purchasing from a non-participating drugstore. As of one month ago I am using a participating drugstore. 4. I don't know if drugs have any bearing on the $150 deductible. 5. Lately, more health care people are aware of the upcoming changes in Military Retiree healthcare. 6. Overall, I like the TSSD program. Will like it better on 10-1-01. P.S. I went to the session held in Longview [Texas] but there wasn't room enough for me (and others) to get in.

- The program has progressed greatly since its implementation. There was a lot of confusion in the beginning.

- I certainly agree strongly with the new "TRICARE for Life" program for all.

- I am glad that TRICARE will become available for all retirees in Oct. '01. If necessary, the current premium I am paying ($1,440) could continue if the overall cost of universal TRICARE places the program in jeopardy due to funding.

- So far we've had excellent results getting prescriptions from VA and Merck-Medicare Services. And it is nice to pay less [of a] premium. Is TRICARE free in October? Will we automatically be switched to the new TRICARE? We so desire.

- The Demonstration Program was a definite improvement over our previous supplemental insurance program, especially in reductions of costs related to drug coverage.

- Excellent plan. Especially the drug program.

- We needed something beyond Medicare for hospital, doctor, and pharmacy costs for major surgery. The demonstration program was timed just right for me.

- I consider TSSD to be a wonderful blessing. Thank You.

- Just keep the TRICARE health program going.

- 1. When I present my TRICARE card at the insurance desk, there is always a "groan" coupled with "CHAMPUS" which must have a bad reputation. I hasten to tell them that TRICARE pays faster than Premier Health, my previous backup insurance! Hope this continues when more retired military join TRICARE! 2. Always happy to immediately pay my TRICARE quarterly payment since it is about [X] of what I used to pay for my policy with Premier Health. 3. Regret that it took Congress so long to "right the wrong"—I don't have much time left to enjoy the benefit!! But others will and they earned it—without paying for it. 4. [Private company/employer] contributes to my prescriptions but their program is limited to a retirement credit of $50,000 and I retired in 198X—What happens when they say that is all used up?

- We are very satisfied with the TRICARE Senior Supplement Demonstration program. It has serviced our needs very well. When will we be eligible for the TRICARE for Life?

- I hope TRICARE Senior Supplement Program will continue in the future. Thanks.

- TRICARE has been a very good program for our family.

- I greatly appreciate the TRICARE Supplement Program. It is a fair and reasonable program for retired military people.

- Before TRICARE Senior there was nothing. Now I think TRICARE Senior is a very good program. I hope it will be permanent and the price will not increase. I feel military health care should be free. But would be willing to contribute to the cost.

- I look forward to 1 Oct. 2001 and no deductibles.

- We are very satisfied with the TSSD program. Everyone at mail order pharmacy and TRICARE SW is so courteous, nice, professional, and helpful. There have been no problems. I have had extensive surgery, medication, hospitalization, and rehab in the past six (6) months with absolute minimum effort and personal expense. The same feeling is for Medicare; they are wonderful.

Comments from Enrollees: Information

- I live 130 miles from nearest military medical facility or hospital and it has been very expensive for me to get medical care and prescriptions. Writing rules and instructions on medical plans must be an exacting challenge. Instructions are oftentimes very ambiguous and unclear in some areas. Those who draft and finalize TRICARE rules and regulations must constantly bear in mind the audience (age group especially) for whom they are writing. Too, a clear, concise, and very lucid manual on the new TRICARE will be a good item for one to have.

- Still am not sure of deductible portion of plan. When does the plan go out? Is it 1 Oct 01 when the plan comes into effect? I do know with getting older we can [anticipate] many health problems and I hope with new health care program coming on we will be covered as promised years ago.

- Would like a more clear picture (options) of what to do after 1 April '01 and 1 Oct '01 (i.e., do I keep TSSD or not after 1 April? after 1 Oct?).

Comments from Enrollees: MTF Care

- I truly miss my days when I could go to a military facility and receive Comprehensive Medical Coverage. After retirement under Medicare, it has been a rat race. From year to year I never seem to have the same doctor, same coverage, same anything. One time Medicare cost is one price, the next it is different. As I grow older it seems that my options are fewer, more complicated, and less helpful. It has become an assembly line to mediocrity.

- The medical service and cost for health care of TRICARE Military Retirees should be returned to military hospitals to save the systems.

- I have used [the] VA hospital facility, Shreveport, LA, for past several years and I am basically satisfied. Some problems—delay in getting appointment, attitude of non-staff personnel (do not answer questions—normal response: "Put card in tray. Have a seat") and parking.

- Prior to the demonstration program, I had to drive 1XX miles one way to Fort Hood, Texas, to get prescriptions filled.

- I retired in 197X. Since I live 1XX miles from the nearest military facility, I found it impossible to utilize their medical facilities. Military dental care was a joke. I did utilize their prescription drugs, but their reorganization about 15 years ago made this impossible. I have been enrolled in the TRICARE Senior

Supplement Demonstration Program since May 2000. This program saved me many dollars on drugs.

Comments from Enrollees: Other Areas

- I signed up for this program for major medical coverage should I become senile or injured (I ride horseback, ski, race a small sailboat, any of which can cause injury) and need long-term expensive care. I have been treated for prostate and lung cancer. Both are now under control (had PSAO.Z). There are no military facilities nearby but I'm close to the Palo Alto VA Hospital—some interaction here would be very helpful. Thank you for asking!

- Since for more than five years all my medical has been at the VA Hospital with them telling me that they do not file with other medical insurance, I could question a need for any other coverage—however, I have continued with coverage. Prior, [I had] same as wife's coverage, now with demo program.

- There has been a mix-up about my spouse's eligibility for coverage.

- 100% of my medical and prescription services needs were and are provided by the local VA (Palo Alto Medical Center, California) facilities and I am very satisfied with same.

- 1. Recognize that TSSD and TFL users are older and can confuse more easily—keep it simple! (Ask [yourself] the question—if I were 85 would it be clear?). 2. Explanation of benefits show TRICARE approved amounts—is this relevant for a supplement policy? 3. Minimize association with CHAMPUS due to its bad reputation in some cases.

- Why are we unable to get civilian [written] prescriptions filled at VA hospitals?

- If TRICARE offered a policy which would cover long-term care at a civilian facility of our choosing at an affordable rate we would be interested.

- My wife has had and is having a lot of medical problems and I am not sure we could have survived while in the military and after I retired had it not been for the medical program.

- I would like to have long-term health care benefits included in the TRICARE program.

- It is my hope that the recently passed bill in Congress that provides "Medical Care for Life" as was implied when I became a career officer will truly come to pass on October of 2001. I do not care for HMOs or the like. A Medicare Supplement like the F Plan with medications would be best.

Comments from Enrollees: Prescription Benefits

- Merck-Medco [NMOP] pharmacy plan is great. [Merck-Medco manages the National Mail Order Pharmacy for TRICARE/DoD.]

- Why is some required medication (e.g., nuclear medication) not covered by Medicare or TRICARE Senior Demonstration? Some of the medications can be given on an outpatient basis but are given on an in-patient status. [Is it because the] medication is by injection??

- Until the Presidio closed some 12 to 15 years ago, we were quite pleased with the medical services we received at Letterman Hospital, San Francisco. We use the military mail order pharmacy program most of the time. This is an outstanding program both from the standpoint of prompt service and cost.

- Why don't you combine drug purchases onto one claim form? Would save a lot of money! I have trouble with CHAMPUS and medication prescriptions refills. They hold up refills on a 30-day supply on the 28th day. When does TRICARE start payments? I am paying out of my pocket.

- TRICARE Demo (Medical) has been very good. Pharmacy part has been unsatisfactory. All contacts with Merck [prescription service] by phone have been very unsatisfactory due to the attitude of customer service personnel. At present time, I have an appeal pending on a drug prescribed by a doctor of medicine. TRICARE said it was "off label." The way I read the pamphlet on the pharmacy plan, I could pay 20% at a participating pharmacy and TRICARE would pay the rest, which they won't do. I had to pay the entire bill for the prescription medicine.

- Would like to have MTF prescription privileges plus TRICARE Senior prescription plan. MTF drugs don't cover enough different drugs but are free [for] what is covered.

Comments from Enrollees: "The Promise"

- I believe the government did not respond to the promise to military retirees who stayed in for the required 20 years [and] they were promised complete medical care. The government only did this when most of us were dead.

- After spending 20 years of my life in the armed forces, I feel the government has let me and a lot of other retirees down by closing bases and medical facilities that were very close that we could use. I also feel the U.S. Government could make it a hell of a lot easier on us if they would not cut allocations for medical needs so Congress can vote themselves more pay that they don't deserve in the first place. We are in dire need of more medical facilities for retirees, not richer congressmen and women.

- Yes, I would like to say that I became an officer from the enlisted and warrant officer ranks. During my time as an enlisted man I was continuously promised free medical care for myself and my wife until the end of our lives. I assume that the new TRICARE program that starts October 1, 2001 is a step in this direction. I would offer that "it is about time."

- I retired after 2X years in the military. I was promised free medical, dental, and optical care for the rest of my life. Now I don't get s——. Other government retirees get all kinds of medical, etc. Life in the military is not rosy—you have to put up with a lot of rotten crap and misery. I did it because I grew up in the 30s (the Depression). I didn't want to end up like my father. He didn't have a pot to piss in and then the Social Security robbed him. I don't understand all the lingo on medical plans. I wish there was some place I could go to and ask questions. I would like to hand over a copy of a plan I have now and ask outright—is this or is it not better than TRICARE?

- TRICARE for Life is what we were promised. Just help make sure it stays on board.

- Thanks for finally fulfilling the promise of medical care for life if you re-up for 20 [years].

- Strongly feel that the Social Security/Government should honor the promise of health care for life to retirees who entered the service prior to 1956. It was a solemn promise and should be kept.

- I enlisted in the U.S. Army Airforce in 194X [and] retired in 196X. I was promised many times—even when I reenlisted—that I would have free medical care for life if I stayed 2X years. This has not been the case. [I have had] no dental [plan] for over 25 years. The [medical program staff] used to act like you were fourth cousins. It is good to see some change. It is really needed financially.

- I earnestly believe it would be fair and proper for the new TRICARE to pick up 100% of medical expenses that Medicare does not pay. Similar to Plan F on other supplementals.

- We live about 1XX miles from the nearest military facility and/or VA hospital. We have never had the opportunity to use a military hospital. I retired from the army in 196X. This is my "first" opportunity to benefit from what we were promised. Thank God!

- I feel that the government broke faith with veterans who gave over twenty years of service and were then excluded from military facilities. The proposed TRICARE for Life in conjunction with Medicare sounds promising but the truth will come out when it is implemented.

- TRICARE for Life and mail order pharmacy program is a *great* step to insure our health care promised to veterans when we enlisted. Please do all you can to promote passage of TFL. Thanks for all you do.

- We are satisfied with the new health rules signed into law for [retirees] 65 and over as [of] 10/01/01 by President Clinton (it's about time).

- TSSD fills a gap that occurred when we reached 65 and were dropped by CHAMPUS. TSSD is a program that offers benefits that I *assumed* would always be there, but were not. I have appreciated the benefits offered by TSSD.

- When I enlisted in the U.S. Navy in 195X, I was promised free medical care for myself and my spouse for rest of [our lives] if I fulfilled a 20-year period of service. That promise has not been kept. I did 2X years of faithful service.

- I served more than 20 years' active service in the U.S. Army. The U.S. Government in turn gave me a written guarantee to provide health care for me and my wife for the remainder of our lives. My government betrayed me and broke their promise. I am enrolled in the TRICARE Senior Demonstration Program for which me and my wife pay a combined total of $196.00 per month plus deductible and copayments. This program is far from acceptable at that cost and I consider it nothing more than a slap in the face.

- Went to Naval Service in 194X—retired 197X—was promised free health care for my dependents and myself—broken at the magic age of 65—resent it! Senators, representatives, nonmilitary federal employees get better [treatment]—why?

- I appreciate having TRICARE Senior Supplement Demonstration for this short period of time since my retirement and welcome the new TRICARE for Life due this year in conjunction with Medicare. I was promised free health care for life each time I enlisted. After 2X years service and 2 wars later, I had to have a supplement to my CHAMPUS and Medicare for 3X years which I should not have had to have, but I will accept [it and] be happy to receive this new health benefit. I just wish it could have came sooner. A lot of my fellow retirees and their families could have enjoyed the health care [peace] of mind. I just hope that nothing happens to sidetrack this any further.

- For the Department of Defense, at this time or ever, to be asking these questions about the Veteran Retirees health care demonstrates they do not remember the promises given to all retirees when they were asked to reenlist, thus convincing the reenlisted to stay in the Military to serve their country. WHY [did they reenlist]? BECAUSE of the benefits [they were] told the reenlisted would be able to give to themselves and/or families even if the military person was killed or disabled. They were also told that they themselves would have full health care no matter what. Never was it told to the reenlisted that when they turned 65, "You will be responsible to buy health care for you and your family to cover the family's medical problems, which will cost you more than two or three months of your retiree's pay."

Comments from Enrollees: Provider Access

- Comments from my cardiologist: Dropped TRICARE because of low reimbursement rates and very slow reimbursements. We are having an increasingly hard time finding practitioners, clinics, and testing facilities that will accept TRICARE because they say [TRICARE] is low [paying] and slow [to] pay.

- Any plan that excludes use of our selected doctors and hospital will not be acceptable to my wife or me.

- My wife's doctor told her that TRICARE pays less than Medicare—33% of bill. Medicare pays 50-75%. How about recommending higher payments? She is unable to go to many doctors and clinics because they won't accept TRICARE.

- Not many program physicians available in our area.

- I eagerly enrolled in the TRICARE SSD program on May 1, 2000. However, when I received all the papers and details, I learned that none of my doctors or my hospital was on the TRICARE network.

- One of my doctors refused to accept this program because of slow payments under the regular TRICARE program.

- Doctors are screening patients to exclude Medicare and government supplement insured individuals.

Comments from Eligibles: Alternative Insurance

- My wife and I are covered by an HMO that has a special contract with my former civilian employer. The premiums deducted from our Social Security checks together with a premium paid by my former employer provide us with fantastic coverage. 1. Office visits—$0 co-pay. 2. Prescriptions—$5 each. 3. ER visit—$20 co-pay.

- My wife and I have used Kaiser health care system for 35 years and have been extremely satisfied. Using my company retirement medical benefits, both my wife (for $93.00 a month) and myself ($50.00 Medicare Part B costs) can remain with Kaiser Permanente medical plan with $10.00 co-pay for each doctor visit and $5.00 (my prescription refill cost) and $10.00 (for my wife's refill) which is very reasonable. Laboratory work and tests require no copay.

- Hope [my survey responses] are okay. They are my thinking on the subject. At my age, one wonders if you should be changing system(s). If we do, it will be the third change.

- I am very disappointed with this plan because it does absolutely nothing for me. Any prescription drug program I have must be used before I can use the less-expensive TRICARE plan. There are no medical facilities in my area.

- We (my wife and I are currently enrolled in TRICARE Dental Coverage [Delta Dental]). If the level of reimbursement for dental services received is any indication of the level of reimbursement we would receive for TRICARE medical services, we feel that we are better off with our current HMO, Kaiser.

- We have not relied upon health care, since my retirement, at any military facility mainly because of the health plans available through my employer (private company). Then with the advent of all the facility closures in the past eight years, we just felt safer with our HMO and carried it into our Medicare A and B plans.

- My spouse has employer benefits which we were able to carry into retirement, including prescription drug benefits. We are very pleased with our benefits under this supplement to the Medicare plan and at this time do not plan on TRICARE enrollment. We are very fortunate to have this coverage, including drugs and doctor preference. Subsequently, as stated above, plan no changes at this time.

- Participation by both my spouse and myself is subsidized by my former employer. It is therefore more economic for us, compared to TRICARE participation costs. Do not live close to any military medical facilities.

- I relied almost exclusively on military health and dental care until the base closure. Now, health care is attended to by FEHBP (at a civilian health care facility). At present, I have no dental coverage as the plan [benefits] are not attractive.

- After retirement in 196X, I entered civilian employment. Regardless of the company, medical and dental benefits were always included at 80%/20%. Never used any military benefits following retirement—just the monthly [pension] check.

- I am currently retired from private enterprise and civil service. I have my own health care insurance. It's very expensive.

- I have always had very good care at the Veterans Hospital in Palo Alto. Have HMO but only used it once for services at El Camino Hospital.

- As a retired military person who was exposed ten times to radiation and was the recipient of a Purple Heart, I qualify to get veterans affairs benefits. There are no available military hospitals in my area. So I am more than grateful to receive VA care.

- The health insurance choices from my civilian retirement are much better than what I currently know about what a military retiree receives. My civilian retirement plan covers all health needs except vision and "long-term care." My cost is $5.00 copay per prescription drug. My HMO covers all costs not handled by Medicare, with very few exceptions. It is great coverage by the State of California for retired teachers—much, much, much better than what I remember about military benefits.

- The VA Hospital is only four miles away, and I have the best care anyone could ever ask for. Thank you.

- We are happy with Kaiser Permanente. It's close to home.

- Generally, I am happy with Kaiser HMO, my wife is also [happy with it]. If we should leave this area that could change. We would then rely more heavily on TRICARE.

- I am a disabled veteran and go to the VA hospital all the time. The VA takes very good care of me and I really appreciate it.

- My spouse and I have excellent coverage by a former civilian employer. We are pleased to have TRICARE as a possible future backup for us.

- We like Kaiser Permanente Senior Advantage. We choose our own doctor, except starting this year we pay a $30 premium each month. Beside what we are paying for Medicare, for myself it costs a little over $500 and my wife pays over $900, which is too much on my wife's part. Kaiser Permanente has everything you need to take care of your health needs.

- My late wife was employed by Kaiser Hospital, which includes full medical coverage for life—dental, prescription, and optical coverage—at no cost.

- Since retirement I've been satisfied with Kaiser.

- Medicare forwards the claim forms directly to my supplementary carrier (TROA Mediplus). No additional paperwork on my part. Mediplus pays to physician the 20% difference after I [pay] the Medicare deductible.

- In addition to my military retirement, I am covered by a retirement plan from private industry. I participate in Kaiser HMO senior advantage and sign over my Medicare Part B and pay a minimal [premium] (less than $10 a month) to my former employer. I am very happy with Kaiser and have never felt motivated to explore military retiree health care alternatives because (1) I suspect that getting it would involve complicated paperwork; (2) I am concerned about where I would need to go to obtain the care, especially considering recent military base closings in Northern California; (3) I value continuity in keeping my personal physician and I assume that rotation of military personnel would jeopardize that situation; (4) I do not know what freedom of physician choice military medical care would offer; at Kaiser I can choose or change my primary care physician and choose from at least 6 or 8 physicians in each of 3 locations which are within a 10-mile radius of my home; and (5) I have several friends who are in Kaiser Senior Advantage and have seen the level of benefits they receive and how satisfied they are with their coverage. IN SUMMARY: Kaiser was there, immediately accessible, and covered by my private industry retirement benefits. Military care had a lot of unknowns and uncertainties. So I chose the easier path. I have been with Kaiser since 199X and have the same primary care physician that I started with. At the same time, I don't want to close any doors to military care in the event that circumstances change. FOR WHAT IT'S WORTH: Even though Kaiser offers a dental program, I have never explored it. I have had my own dentist since 198X and pay his full fees with no insurance assistance. Right now I can afford him and think he is worth it.

- Kaiser has an excellent health plan.

- Our HMO costs about the same as TRICARE.

- I am retired from [state employer] and both of our health [plans], including dental coverage, are furnished by the [State] Retirement System and we are very satisfied with our health insurance coverage.

- When military facilities became unavailable to me I joined Kaiser Senior Advantage. It has been a very satisfactory, low-cost alternative for me and my wife. And the Kaiser Hospital is located within two miles of my home.

- The VA in Palo Alto, California, has taken great care of me for a long time.

- We have a Medicare supplement plan provided by my former employer. For a reasonable cost to me, it provides good coverage for routine medical care. [With our] past experience with HMOs and military medical care, we foresee relying on care which is outside of our central [area] and may not be available when we need it. Unfortunately, we did not expect that to be the case when we "signed on" way back. TRICARE may be a step in correcting the wrong, but if it comes, it must be reliable.

- The current proposed "TRICARE for Life" cannot compare to the current coverage I have with a federal employer's health plan. To my knowledge there is no coverage for dental care. It appears to me that there is co-payment for medication whereas under my current federal coverage I am restricted to a copayment of $2 per prescription. Who concocted this plan? According to my California senators, there are elements within retiree organizations, such as [respondent named an individual associated with TROA], that instead of working for retiree issues are only interested in their own personal high-paid job.

- My wife and I are now enrolled in Secure Horizons but the cost has gone up. We have had military care in the past and have been very happy with the doctors and the prescription benefits. We would prefer to have military medical care. Thanks for your survey.

- Prior to qualifying for Medicare, my total out-of-pocket expense was 20% of covered charges. Since Medicare, the VA charges me $50 per visit and my secondary pays nothing until my out-of-pocket [expenses] to Medicare exceed $2,000!!

- I plan to drop my HMO (Secure Horizons) on September 30, 2001, and use Medicare with TRICARE for Life as a supplement. Also, [I plan to use] the mail order pharmacy beginning April 2001.

- I enrolled in TRICARE but could not use it because I was on an HMO—Secure Horizon.

- Very satisfied with the supplement USAA Health Care except for prescription drugs [coverage].

- As an 8X-year-old widower living alone and in reasonable health, Medicare and my copay retirement health plan from my former civilian employment are [providing] satisfactory coverage for my medical needs at a very reasonable cost. Unless there is some noteworthy change in my present health care coverage, I feel no need for any additional health care assistance. That was my reason for not participating in this survey at your initial mailing.

- With a 20% medical retirement, I have been accepted in a VA clinic within 30 miles of my current home. But if my wife has to have medical care, we must go to our family doctor, which took two years to be accepted due to lack of qualified doctors. We are now both being accepted for medical needs at a civilian facility in another town which accepts Medicare and which files our medical bills with the medical supplement insurance company. As long as we can continue in this program, we are satisfied, but it would be nice to be able to join a supplemental insurance plan which would be less expensive each month.

- The Senior Program as I understood it was fairly expensive with lots of hassles with doctors, claims, etc. We have a personal M.D. that we both like and the USAA Supplement . . . the Medicare claims go directly to USAA and leave us completely out of the "paper" loop. We get all our medications (long-term maintenance) at the military pharmacy—90 days' [supply] at a time—so this is no real inconvenience. With the new benefit coming April 1 for the NMOP, our bases are covered. Also with TRICARE becoming second payer in October 2001, that will enable me to cancel my private Medigap plans. Just hope they keep it "funded"!

- I retired from [public employer]. Part of my retirement benefits is health benefits with drug [coverage] and copayment. I have no information on the TRICARE cost of anything.

- I am service-connected disabled to receive all my care from the VA.

- We could not afford to drop current insurance if we could not be reinstated after the demonstration since we would have a problem getting any plan, from any company, if we had canceled.

- My wife and I are both covered by Medicare, Parts A and B. Also, we are covered by BC/BS of Texas. We have not used military facilities since I retired.

- 1. Our nearest military medical facility is more than 100 miles away. 2. Fortunately, we have sufficient money to fill the gaps after Medicare and my former company insurance program pays [for our care].

- With Medicare and the [employer supplement], we both have excellent coverage and will continue to have it with the death of either of us. Others are not so fortunate.

- We would very much appreciate having TRICARE if we were not already enrolled in a civilian health care plan of our previous employer.

- We are both military retired and disabled. We both use the VA clinics and hospital only. Some of these questions don't apply to us because we use the VA. For about X years we used Barksdale AFB, Louisiana, and were told we could not use it anymore because we live over 4X miles from the facility.

- 1. How about long-term care? Nursing home care? 2. How about prescriptions?

- It seems the military drops the retired from medical (CHAMPUS) when it is most needed and a veteran must wait a long time for help from the VA. The prescription drugs from base have been a big help.

- The VA says that I am not eligible for medical care.

- I have insurance from employment after retiring from the USAF. My insurance is paid by the state and I must pay for my spouse's. My only problem with this private (group) insurance is the deductible and co-insurance. The prescription insurance with my group insurance is a lifesaver even though the co-payment has increased almost annually. The loss of TRICARE at age 65 has hurt but the reinstatement of prescription [benefits] after age 65 will be helpful.

- I am retired from [public employer]. They pay for my Blue Cross/Blue Shield supplemental insurance and I carry my wife on the same policy. That may affect some of my answers.

- When my wife and I reached age 65 our health insurance with CHAMPUS stopped. We had to purchase supplemental insurance to pick up charges after Medicare. This currently costs approximately $1,200.00 annually for each of us and does not cover medicine. TRICARE will be a great help to us.

- I have very good insurance which I [pay for] on a bank draft. Haven't thought of TRICARE. My supplement pays everything. I pay only for a few drugs. [I may be interested] if [the program] is properly made to [my] satisfaction. My eyesight is very bad and [there is] no one to read it to me.

- On my only approach to a VA medical facility I was told that I was ineligible for services because of my income. I am a retired service member with 80% disability.

- Medicare Parts A and B and private Medigap (although expensive) have taken care of us pretty well. We are in the boondocks (isolated area) away from military medical facilities. Would especially like Rx medicines at reduced costs.

- My experience with VA facilities leaves much to be desired. This is due to the attitude of some personnel and poor English-speaking ability on the part of medical personnel (physicians).

- We started TSSD 01 April '01. Before that, we were in Medigap Plan F. It cost a bit over $3,000.00 per year. Prescriptions (when available) came from BAFB, Louisiana—2XX miles round trip.

- I am 100% permanently service-connected disabled and my wife or another person needs to drive me 1XX miles to Waco for dental care. I also need a doctor after the clinic (VA) hours sometimes and have to pay for care at a local doctor's office or hospital. I need 100% care from my wife and she is worked down all the time taking care of me. I have to pay for Medicare and Blue Cross/Blue Shield supplemental insurance to cover this. Also, if I need drugs I have to pay for them because I don't have time to order them by mail.

- I am waiting to see how this new [TFL] is going to turn out before dropping my insurance supplement. Will be glad when it all becomes effective as the supplement we have now is very expensive and seems to go up every year. Plus there are no medical benefits.

Comments from Eligibles: Claims Processing

- I think any system that is introduced should keep administration and paper work at a definite minimum.

- Since "TRICARE for Life" will be secondary to Medicare, it is *most* important that the effort in submitting secondary documentation be minimized! Use plastic ID cards so paperwork can be zero! Increase number of authorized pharmacies/chains. Thank you.

- Linking Medicare payments to TRICARE would simplify our payment process and reduce our records significantly.

- Based on experience with CHAMPUS/TRICARE in the years prior to reaching age 65, my spouse and I do not have much faith in TRICARE claims being handled quickly and expeditiously.

- One of the main problems with the over-65 TRICARE is the failure to authorize automatic rollover from Medicare-approved changes unless additional paperwork is forwarded by the person/agency rendering service. Such action is not only a burden to [the] user but expands the bureaucracy and increases the cost of the program. Nearly all Medigap coverage authorizes a rollover.

- Few of us have Xerox machines. This makes an onerous chore out of record-keeping and form-filling requirements. During the last months of life, we will normally not be capable of [doing] any paperwork. The caregivers (doctors, hospitals, etc.) are all doing the claim filing now. Let them continue [to do so] as this is only an additional "supplemental policy."

Comments from Eligibles: Cost/Coverage

- [TSSD is] too expensive. This is only a pilot program and if not continued permanently we could not then reenroll in our Medigap program.

- Would like to have medical coverage overseas.

- Our military medical insurance (supplement) should be at no cost.

- The literature sent by the military never says anything about coordination of benefits.

- Some questions that arise regarding TRICARE: I am an AF retiree—7X years of age—in fair health. If I enroll in TRICARE, do I keep my HMO plus all its benefits? From information I have received so far from TRICARE, some costs are percentages of total bills (i.e., hospital plus drugs)—this is "questionable" as to total costs. In my opinion, retirees 65 and older need clearer information as to coverage—the costs and availability.

- At age 65, I decided not to participate in Medicare B. I'm now 8X. I'd like to get some low-cost prescription drug coverage without having to pay back-premium penalties to Medicare. If TRICARE had some exception to being a Medicare participant, I'd be interested even at double the rates for Medicare recipients. Otherwise, I'll continue paying for all medical costs out of my own pocket.

- I plan to retire from my present occupation and to travel overseas, possibly to retire permanently outside the United States. To be eligible for health care benefits for routine, nonemergency treatment outside the United States would be important to me. Above all, I would be reluctant to enroll in any health care plan that would require me to become ineligible for treatment in U.S. military hospitals overseas or in the United States.

- Cannot see any advantages compared to our present coverage. Do not need the extra hassle after being exempted (pushed out) from care we earned by our service to our country. [Respondent noted paperwork, cost, travel, and finding new primary care as other decisionmaking factors.].

- Need a dental and eye care plan. There is no low-cost dental or eye care plan in this county.

- I am interested in long-term care.

- How about Dental Care? My teeth were [damaged] while in the military. [Dental care] cost me around $10,000 in the past 10 years or so. TRICARE dental stinks. I'm in it [and] they deduct [it] from my pay, but it doesn't cover anything to speak of.

- It is my understanding TRICARE doesn't cover everything MEDICARE covers. If TRICARE only covers certain items, then this not a MEDICARE Supplement.

- Need to be provided with more assistance with prescription drugs.

- I feel like as a retiree, I should have the same benefits on Medicare as I had with CHAMPUS prior to reaching 65.

- I believe that the cost will be far above the health services received.

- I was interested in military insurance but it costs more than outside premiums. I had to change over. Hope this TRICARE will come into effect. That will save funds for the retirees.

- My only comment—Upon retirement, I thought I would have better medical coverage, but at age 65 I went under Medicare which doesn't provide drugs. A complicated process that confronts a 7X-year-old—with all these plans, Medicare A and B, TRICARE, supplemental plans, etc., it is sometimes confusing.

- We make about $2X,000 a year and cannot afford a health insurance plan.

- I have no other insurance coverage as the cost is much greater than I can afford due to the high cost of living. I do appreciate someone is stepping in and showing some concern for the retirees. I have a bad back from military [service] and still hold a full-time job to live and do not know when, if ever, I will be able to quit. Thanks again for trying.

- They need a supplemental policy that will cover the Medicare and hospital deductible at a reasonable cost.

Comments from Eligibles: General

- My pre-Medicare experience with TRICARE was frustrating. Bureaucracy was stifling! Needed constant phone calls to get authorization for any contact with specialists. TRICARE pay was so low and [they expected] doctor's staff to handle so much minutia with health care finders at TRICARE that no good doctors would stay [in the plan]. The result was a frequent search for a competent physician. In the vernacular, "IT SUCKED"!

- I remember when many doctors would not accept new CHAMPUS/Medicare patients. What happens if TRICARE is dropped by Congress? What happens if the selected TRICARE doctor is inconveniently far away? I am not sure TRICARE would be any different from my present HMO, which is primarily a Henry Ford mass-production process.

- I do not like TRICARE for Life!! Reasons: no dental coverage, no eye exam or glasses coverage, no annual physical coverage, immunizations not covered, hearing exam and hearing aids not covered. I belong to Secure Horizons at $55 per month with all the above included. To join the retiree dental plan (and my wife also) is $68 a month. We have no other worries—we just go to the doctor and get great service. Having used CHAMPUS, I guess I am saying, "I don't trust TFL to be there when I need it."

- Would like to continue in current HMO with TRICARE taking care of copays and monthly charges.

- We enrolled in TRICARE Dental only. Found it to be poor coverage for the cost.

- I am still working and will continue to do so as long as my health permits. I don't know when, but when I'll be at that age, will I be eligible to join TRICARE?

- I hope that one of the goals we seek is to eliminate double and even triple sources of medical coverage (i.e., Medicare and TRICARE and flight care, etc.). Anytime you have paperwork flowing to and from more than one source there's bound to be problems.

- In three years when my wife reaches age 65 and joins Medicare, I will re-evaluate my decision to join TRICARE.

- Took advantage of base medical facilities until [I was] kicked out at age 65. [Took advantage of] pharmacy usage until facility closed. Have retired employee medical and pharmacy coverage [otherwise] I would join TRICARE or like coverage. Did not get the free medical care after age 65.

- Waiting with some skepticism as to just how good the TRICARE program for retirees will work out. Examples: Will doctors accept the plan? How effective will the prescription drug program be?

- Looking forward to "TRICARE For Life" full program!!!

- We would rather have military-sponsored health care.

- TRICARE offers nothing I do not have at this time except paperwork aggravation and the lack of dependability of any federal program.

- I believe TRICARE could be set up similar to an HMO-type [plan] (Secure Horizons). So you could see your local doctors and hospitals when needed. I might be interested in that type of plan. Also, the lower cost of prescription drugs would be beneficial. Thank you. Hope this can help.

- Temporary nature of the program was a primary concern. I attended a seminar when the program was first offered. Also, we like Palo Alto medical clinic, which has a full staff of doctors and is only one mile from home. Proximity of Stanford hospital also important if needed. Military health care is not an option. All medical facilities in military bases have closed in our area. Nearest military base with medical staff is 8X miles away. I have used the VA hospital in the past, which is X miles from home, but I earn too much and must pay $50 per visit and $800 for overnight hospitalization. If senior TRICARE is on a permanent basis, I would reconsider. The TRICARE program we used when we were under 65 worked fine. Cost would have to be less than half the $150 monthly we now pay and ideally would include the Palo Alto medical clinic. Also, having to go through a primary care doctor to get to a specialist is cumbersome. Neither plan we have requires primary care doctor permission to see a specialist, not even my HMO. I remember being told as a young person that a reason to stay in the service was the medical facilities available in retirement. Now, all bases are closed. I am glad to see continued interest in medical care for retired service personnel.

- I'm covered by Kaiser for everything, but it costs me a monthly fee for myself and my wife. How about kicking in a little to help the coverage and prescriptions?

- In my opinion, Military Health Care for the retirees is a tragic joke. My friends also share this feeling.

- My recommendation is: TRICARE should pay the 20% deductible under Part B of Medicare. Also, Medicare should provide a drug benefit plan for retired military (and dependents). Annual deductible for this prescription drug benefit should be $100 for each person.

- I am satisfied with the care I (we) receive with the Medicare/military support coupled with the supplemental insurance we have purchased. Change to TRICARE would have to [at] a minimum maintain (a) level of care and (b) level of costs. My only concern is that the support I receive from the military pharmacy will not [cover] the drugs prescribed by my civilian doctor. The support I receive at this time is absolutely outstanding (FREE).

- We are very grateful for the TRICARE for Life program and will use it when it is available.

- 1. Military facilities are not always within traveling distance. 2. Paperwork is just too much. Drives us nuts! 3. Whatever program you do needs to be SIMPLE!!

- My wife is enrolled in TRICARE, I was enrolled but taken off when I turned 65. My wife and myself look forward to being eligible for TRICARE Senior Supplement later this year when we both are 65.

- Instructions should be simple as 1-2-3. The military system is unreliable for medical care—programs are always changing. The answer is simple—just provide free medical care as promised and reduce the administration.

- TRICARE for Life as I understand it will provide relatively inexpensive prescriptions starting April 1, 2001, and Medicare supplemental starting October 1, 2001. If this is true and is funded, it's about time.

- Instead of this exercise here, we have always believed the military should have the same good coverage as federal employees and Congressmen.

- Medical paperwork is a definite deterrent to me!! Our pharmacy plan keeps going up on what we have to pay. TRICARE wasn't selected because we don't know how it affects our civilian medical plan by employer. We have major medical for hospital [care]. Does TRICARE offer this? After 3X years in the Navy, I have received no medical help after turning 65. Nearest facility is 1XX miles away. They do not treat retirees. I feel betrayed by my government. They promised free health care to me and my spouse for life and haven't kept their promise. TRICARE is at least a step in the right direction!

- 1. We are looking forward to TRICARE for Life effective 1 Oct. 2001 (would like to have it sooner). 2. We are looking forward to low-cost prescriptions effective 1 Apr 2001. 3. I was not sure at all if I would be approved for insurance with a civilian insurance company after the demonstration time period ended. 4. The Demonstration Program appeared to me as being more expensive than my current supplement that I have for Medicare.

- I am looking forward to the TRICARE for Life in October and the pharmacy advantages in April.

- I look forward to the new TRICARE program.

- We had a town hall meeting conducted by TRICARE. The person they selected to travel from Washington was bitter, hard to understand, and did not need to be in the employment of the government. We looked up the nearest M.D. that would take TRICARE and his answer was "No." I do not need to enroll in TRICARE Senior Supplement and be treated as a second-class citizen. I don't think you can sell this policy in this area.

- Need choice of hospital and doctor. Do not need to be "hassled" about claims, or [told] no [payment would be made] if [we go to the] wrong doctor or hospital, etc. Need reasonable costs. We don't want a free ride, but an affordable benefits package. Got to get more hospitals and doctors on board!!

Comments from Eligibles: Information

- Don't fully understand the program.

- Since the Army abandoned Northern California, there are no readily available military medical facilities for me. . . . They [were] convenient before then.

- I feel that somehow my wife and I are not as well informed as I would like. Maybe I should become active in some of the retiree programs.

- We did not have enough information to make a decision.

- Medicare/Mediplus meets our needs.

- Just recently received information on the TRICARE Senior pharmacy program, but as of this date I have not received any information on any participating doctors.

- I believe the program should be more widely disseminated and thoroughly explained to retired military (by telephone, fax, etc.).

- I would like to know all about TRICARE, DEERS, and any other insurance for health care.

- We need to compare the costs of our present HMO with the proposed TRICARE, which we are eligible for in Oct. 01 and have to consider both before we change. We are trying to get additional info to weigh the benefits! Also, is prescription coverage a sure thing yet in Medicare? It's still in the Congress!! We are afraid to drop our present coverage before we can "test" the military's!! We are in our 80s and need better care and attention. How far we have to go is another factor and how competent the VA care will be [is another]. We waited six hours one time for a visit!!

- From what little information I had, I did not think I was eligible to join TRICARE.

- Have not received any info on TRICARE as of yet.

- I have received no information about the TRICARE Senior Supplement Demonstration Program other than it exists and is temporary. I will not give favorable consideration to any temporary program. What little information I've been able to obtain indicates that the DoD is still trying to figure out how it should operate. As long as Congress refuses to pay for it, it will never come to fruition, and this "study" will be meaningless.

- Please send us all the information about the TRICARE program—the different options offered and the health insurance premiums or cost per family of two. We would like to choose our own doctor even if we pay a reasonable low-cost monthly premium. Today, most of the physicians are "only" taking patients PPO (EPO or whatever these options are named). It is difficult for patients with HMOs to choose a physician.

- 1. Dental care for military retirees is completely inadequate. 2. TRICARE apparently will not be available for military retired until the latter part of 2001. 3. Information on nursing home facilities for military retired dependents would be beneficial.

- Is there any long-term disability care available for retired military persons and their families?

- Plain, simple, clear information on this and related plans/programs is needed. I get quite confused by the letters, brochures, and pamphlets that are mailed. There must be a way for this program to be properly explained to military retirees.

- What is the difference between Standard TRICARE and Senior TRICARE? Also, [what is the difference] in price? What about psychiatric care? What can TRICARE do for me in comparison with Kaiser Permanente? How are our co-payments determined? Should give more information on this. Will we forfeit our Medicare and have to pay for TRICARE too?

- I have never received an application to join TRICARE. And I have never received instructions on how to enroll.

- I really do not know if TRICARE would be better or not. I don't know the total cost to me. I know I now pay Part B plus $30.00 a month for senior advantage and a copay for drugs.

- Most of my health care is from the VA hospital and I am also using an HMO outside for immediate health care because the hospital is a distance from my home. Please advise me on the possibility of TRICARE.

- I'm not sure we really know enough about the TRICARE Senior Supplement Demo Program to make any evaluation of its value to us.

- We didn't know about this TRICARE. When Moffett Field was shut down, they took our health care away from us.

- I think if we were able to see and talk to people, we might feel that we could use the military services. Prescriptions are hurting us very much [financially] for [my wife's] needs. I wish there was a way we could get more information about who and where we could go to for help and assistance.

- Am not aware of the "TRICARE" program. Desire facilities near home and would not travel excessive distances. Would use civilian facilities, if available, under auspices of TRICARE.

- We don't understand how TRICARE would interact or supplement the Medicare present insurance or location of facilities. Why does the Veterans Administration try to compete with Medicare? Why not [offer] something that Medicare doesn't cover, such as discounted long-term nursing home or home health care? Or partial payment on or tax-deductible long-term care insurance? Although I could be considered affluent in any part of the U.S. but here (SF Bay Area), we have difficulty with occasional small tasks, moving furniture, minor repairs. It would be nice if there was an organization that could send us help for a reasonable cost.

- TRICARE has not been fully explained to us. We are presently undecided if we want to join and when, where, and how we can receive treatment.

- I request you direct us to the TRICARE Senior Supplement program [information]. I should mention that along with others on retired military payroll, effective 1 April 2001, the wife and I can get pharmaceutical needs free at military facilities and at private drug stores. Thanks again.

- How does the military health package, including [the one for] retirees, compare with that of the Federal Civil Service and the one provided to members of Congress?

- I retired from the U.S. Army Reserves after 2 years active duty and 2X years in the Reserves. I was told at one time that I was not eligible for TRICARE ([by] a friend who is a 20-year full-time naval officer, retired also). If I am eligible, I would like to enroll.

- I don't know if I am enrolled in TRICARE and would like to know if I am enrolled.

- 1. Would like more info about TRICARE Senior Supplement Demonstration program. 2. If doctor or hospital charges more than Medicare assigned fees, will TRICARE pay remainder after Medicare and supplemental are paid their allowable amount? 3. If a service is not covered by Medicare, such as an annual physical exam, will TRICARE cover the cost? 4. Must a claim be submitted to Medicare first? 5. Does TRICARE cover travel outside of U.S.?

- It appears the TRICARE benefits coming in October may provide us with more flexibility and choice. In this regard, I would like a more comprehensive explanation of what it's all about and what one must do to join.

- Need more information about TRICARE.

- I need more information about TRICARE Senior Supplement—what does it cover? What does it cost? What are the benefits? How and when do I join?

- I am not acquainted with TRICARE.

- We have no info to compare TRICARE with Medicare A and B or combination of A and B and Blue Cross-Blue Shield.

- I'm not sure that I understand all of the facets of TRICARE. I am most thankful for the promise of the 1 Oct 2001 health care by the VA.

- Would like more information on Senior Supplement Demonstration program. Got very little information about this.

- I do not recall being offered enrollment in any military or government program demonstration or otherwise. Although my wife and I have some limited prescription drug coverage, our out-of-pocket costs for drugs are the largest expenses we have by far. We are very concerned about the cost of longer-term health care (nursing home care).

- What would happen to our present coverage of Medicare A and B, and the group policy from place of retirement that now acts as a supplement that we do not have to pay for? If we have to pay for insurance coverage with the military coverage, how else could the TRICARE policy from the military benefit help us? We don't know enough about this proposal to make an informed decision.

- We don't know anything about TRICARE, but would like to.

- This is all a bunch of confusing, political b——s——. There is no way to understand the benefits.

- My question is, if I join TRICARE Senior, which I have nothing to sign up for, will I be able to go to a physician locally or will they be listed 100 miles from my address? The only information I have is a letter and booklet. Need list of physicians and hospitals—just like TRICARE Prime issued. Thank You.

- Do not know about TRICARE.

- I assumed that TRICARE would link me to a Military Medical Facility. The closest is 1XX miles away. I have been well cared for with Medicare and my TROA Supplement.

- I have to pay for my VA medical. I pay $2 per month per each prescription. I only have heard that TRICARE is great. I've heard that TRICARE is free. I've been led to believe TRICARE will pay that which Medicare doesn't pay. Does TRICARE pay for eyeglasses? Does TRICARE pay the 1-90 day cost of the hospital [stay]?

- Why were we not contacted about this program before now?

- I really appreciate this survey. We have fought for several years to get our military health care back. I am 7X years old and widowed on a fixed income. I can sure use this break. I don't know how to use it, yet (1 OCT 01). I have one question: My present care provider, civilian, has been serving CHAMPUS patients for several years, and me, since 1992. At that time, Barksdale AFB kicked me out. I still get medicine there. How do my provider and the clinic become eligible to participate in the TRICARE program? Thanks.

- I don't know anything about this TRICARE PROGRAM.

- We need to have this program explained in detail, as we haven't understood it yet. Also, I would not like to change not knowing if the program would last and having to start all over with another insurance at 8X years old. We don't live close to any military posts, hospitals, or any other military [facility].

- My supplement to Medicare is under the FEHBP. Will the TRICARE be part of the FEHBP?

- I do not really know what TRICARE is. I have never heard anyone discuss or explain the purpose of TRICARE. No one has ever asked me if I desired to join or participate. This is all a mystery to me.

- I live over 2XX miles from a military base with a hospital. Am at this time not on any hospital rolls, so we could use them. Also the information on TRICARE Senior Supplement has been very sketchy. No cost data—how and what would be covered, etc.?

- With TRICARE: 1. Does our ID card serve as a TRICARE card? 2. Does Medicare forward to TRICARE for payment? 3. Does TRICARE pay what Medicare does not pay? 4. Any deductibles?

- I live approximately 8X miles from an MTF and am really out of the mainstream. There were adequate briefings on TRICARE but health options precluded attendance.

- I am assuming being enrolled in DEERS automatically enrolls [me] into the [TSSD] plan. Although have not been able to use it yet.

- We are supposed to receive the 100% care we were promised in Oct. 2001— why hasn't anyone contacted us?

- We have private supplemental coverage. TRICARE is on a three-year plan??? Then what happens?

- I have never understood this plan—and still don't.

- I feel that there are a great number of people in this area who do not realize they are eligible for the TRICARE demonstration program. I will tell all I know [about it] but someone needs to make a mass mailing and say, hey, you are eligible for the program. I personally think it will be great. Thank you.

Comments from Eligibles: MTF Care

- Free medical and dental service for me and for my spouse was a contractor benefit that encouraged my selecting 2X years of military service as a career. TRICARE could very well prevent BREACH OF CONTRACT. HMOs are not working. I've tried Secure Horizon first and am presently with Kaiser—both are (a) understaffed for services as simple as annual physicals and (b) costly for drugs, eye care, hearing aids, and monthly [fees] due over and above Social Security Medicare A and B charges, etc. ($40 each for myself and wife after moving [to an HMO]). Relief is badly needed in dental care. Kaiser Medicare HMO dropped dental care as part of their inclusive program. [It is now] a separate expense to seniors for dental which offers very little relief under the present so-called discount cost for dental services.

- When I was in the U.S. Navy, they told me to "stay in" and I "would be taken care of medically." And that would be one of my retirement benefits. I found out shortly after I got out, you get very few benefits. It was almost impossible to get into a military hospital or clinic, and when you turned 65 you were dropped like a bad potato.

- I wish there was a military facility closer to me so I could use it.

- I was wounded twice and in a military hospital over two months in 194X. I retired from the Reserves at age 6X and am receiving medical care mostly from the VA and have been in the hospital several times, especially in recent years. I was disappointed that the Navy hospital in Oakland closed. The VA has been good to me but I wish the Navy was still in the area.

- We live in the Greater San Jose Area and are unaware of any military medical facilities close by that are available—and at the same time how we could utilize them if they were available.

- Kaiser is the best thing that has happened to our family of seven children. We lost all of our military bases in our area; before they were closed we got free prescriptions.

- The distance to the nearest military health facility is approximately 7X miles from my home.

- Preferred alternative for both myself and my spouse is health care in military medical facilities (as promised upon entry into service).

- Both my wife and I are well pleased and satisfied with services given to us by [our provider] at Travis AF Base, California.

- With the closure of many military bases (all services), the medical care declined. [With] the reduction of military forces, many of the medical services also were lost. One has to use outside medical personnel with highly trained skills, such as ophthalmologists and hematologists. These specialists are not available at some military installation these days. In the area where I reside, the military bases are CLOSED. Therefore, it is much easier to use civilian medical doctors. VA clinics are located many miles away and not convenient to arrive at. Now, many military bases serve only active duty personnel and their dependents. Retired personnel must wait a long time for an appointment. If they are lucky, the military medical faculty is serving retired service personnel.

- The U.S. government closed down the U.S. Army Letterman Hospital, Oak Knoll Navy Hospital, Moffett Navy Dispensary, all facilities I used for medical care. Meanwhile, the U.S. government was spending millions of dollars building and enlarging the VA hospital in Palo Alto. Closing the U.S. Navy Moffett Field Pharmacy was a disaster, financially and for convenience' sake. Taking care of my 5XX prescriptions by mail with the VA hospital takes more of my time than servicing my investments. The parking lot and design of the VA hospital at Palo Alto is designed for athletes. They use golf cart taxis to get patients from the parking lots to the numerous buildings.

- Due to base closures, there are no military facilities within a three- to four-hour drive.

- When I joined the ROTC in 195X and entered the service in 195X, I was told that medical care in retirement would be free. And so I put in the years until retirement doing all that was asked of me—my part of the bargain/agreement. I feel that the government has failed me and all the other service personnel who now must pay for TRICARE, co-pay, medicines, or whatever. They also say that retirees and reservists are an important part of our military—what if they threw a war and folks refused to go unless the government lived up to its promises? My spouse is employed with Kaiser HMO coverage. My Kaiser Permanente [plan] is cheaper and more convenient. There is no copay on medicines.

- During my retirement, there has not been an available, convenient, or consistent military health care center.

- It's a shame they closed all the clinics and hospitals for the military so all the people in Washington, D.C., can make a name for themselves.

- All of the military bases have been closed in this area; there are no prescription-filling pharmacies. We are unable to drive and it presents a difficulty with no local military bases.

- The military health care facilities that we utilized in the past were closed about ten years ago, namely Oak Knoll Naval Hospital in Oakland, California. The medical facilities at Moffett Air Station in Mountain View, California, were also closed.

- When I retired, there were adequate military facilities available to provide the medical support necessary for my dependent and myself. I have no quarrel with the necessity to reduce these facilities in a peacetime environment; however, Congress should have done something to provide some relief to this sudden loss. The military has done everything to try to take care of its own. My distrust of Congress is the reason I have not enrolled in the TRICARE test program and I've heard no experts on how successfully the test program is progressing.

- I retired from the Army 4X years ago. Moved to the Bay Area in San Francisco. Got good medical service for a while. But then they closed most of all the bases. What few are left are too far away for this 8X-year-old to get to. Luckily, my employer pays most if not all of my health care. I can't even get any service from the VA.

- The closest military base (Travis) is over two hours away—very difficult to plan on military support [for health care].

- In 196X I was told by the administrative office, U.S. Naval Hospital Oak Knoll (Oakland, California) that funds were decreased (the budget) and to go it alone! Meaning that pharmacy and hospital services would not be available for me or my family.

- At present, no military [bases] in the area—all closed down.

- I still resent being arbitrarily shut out by the closing of a nearby military hospital in 1988, which had given excellent treatment to me and my wife for 4X years.

- At present we are only reenrolled at Barksdale for the DEERS program. We have not been to use the doctors, pharmacy, or hospital as of yet. Once and if the program is funded and retirees and spouses are privy to the facilities, I would be happy to fill out any questions you may want to know about the system.

- Nearest military facility is 6X miles away. It's time consuming to get and keep appointments there. Also, there are delays in getting prescriptions filled. Have excellent health for my age and 30-plus years of military service. Therefore, have not used military facilities and the VA is very unsatisfactory!

- I did not know that we could receive our medication free from a military base until one year ago. Since Medicare and our supplemental insurance did not pay for any medication, our medication since turning 65 had cost us approximately $4,000.00 each year for the previous three years. Thank You.

- I live about 5X miles from a military hospital. The time or two I have asked about eye or dental appointments, I was informed they were too busy with active-duty persons and their families. I gave 3X years and believe I deserve military health care. Thank You.

- Live over 8X miles from Shreveport and Barksdale AFB. With TRICARE, could we use local doctors in Gladewater and Longview, Texas?

- I am just looking forward to Oct. 1, 2001, when my spouse and I will be enrolled in the TRICARE for Life program, as the closest military facility (Barksdale AFB) will not treat retirees and their dependents.

- The fact that we have to drive 1XX miles each way to get our prescriptions filled at a military installation is a great inconvenience as well as being a hardship on us. My husband enlisted from here and he should have the same medical benefits as the men who enlisted from towns near the military bases (no equality). We need TRICARE doctors in our area.

- I live 1XX miles from a military medical facility. Made use of pharmacy, outpatient, and clinic service when space is available and it's becoming a long waiting list. Perhaps TRICARE may be desirable in future.

- Because of the distance involved (1XX miles) we do not go to a military installation. Note—I am pleased that someone is finally taking an interest in the older retirees.

- We live too far from a military base to get care there. Being able to get medications at a military base is helpful. Being able to get medication for short-term problems at a local pharmacy would be helpful. Being able to see a physician of choice is helpful. Who wants to drive 25 or 30 miles when ill?

- We used the military hospitals' health care until age 65 and prefer that. [The MTF] made so many changes from month to month that we never knew what to expect next and feared being cut out. We could not depend on it when we needed it.

- Return our health and medical [care] to military hospitals as it was, prior to the downsizing by the last administration in Washington.

- We live about 1XX miles from the nearest military medical facility. Age prevents travel to a military treatment facility.

- We live too far from a military base.

- I am most thankful for those prescriptions available through the military pharmacy, for without them I could not have afforded all the prescribed medications. The items that I must purchase locally are only a minor portion of those that I take daily. Although the medical care I received at the military base prior to 199X was very good, I would not, due to age and distance, care to have to rely on military treatment facilities for my health care.

- I have tried a few times to get help from the Army with no help. The way I could get help was go to Brooks [AFB] in San Antonio; no help on prescriptions from local pharmacy.

- Most of the medications taken by me and my wife are not carried by the pharmacy at the military facility that we would use.

- Would have used military health care facilities . . . except [that I] was cut . . . or denied care at Barksdale AFB, Louisiana.

- I was put out of a military hospital because I live 4X miles from the base.

- [The nearest military health facility is] too great a distance for me to travel due to my declining health. Each visit to the base, I was "talked down to" like I wasn't fit to take up their time. I informed them that they too would be in my place one day. At age 65 and loosing CHAMPUS, we were forced to file bankruptcy due to medical expenses.

- We live too far from the closest military base for it to be practical to use the military to get treatment, but we plan on using the TRICARE mail order drugs.

- I feel it is totally unfair that I should be penalized for: (1) living outside the service zone for TRICARE and (2) having a second payer to Medicare. This makes me ineligible for the mail pharmacy program (especially when I'm now paying $20 copay to the same provider, Merck-Medco!). (3) Finding it often difficult to obtain military care living where I am with chronic, life-shortening service-connected illnesses.

Comments from Eligibles: Other Areas

- Even when we could use CHAMPUS we didn't. In 3X years of marriage we used CHAMPUS for one cesarean operation. We paid medical expenses out of pocket in order to choose our own M.D.'s who were more experienced than the military M.D.'s.

- I have been too ill to read the info sent to me.

- After retirement from the AF I used the facilities at Moffett Naval Air Station. Then Moffett Naval Air Station closed. I used the [private employer] retirement plan for my medical program. I will evaluate the TRICARE Plan and choose the best plan for me and my family. Thanks for the evaluation.

- 1. The distance between you and the doctor or medical facility [is important]. 2. Is "health care" part of our retirement or something we supplement with premiums? 3. The right health plan is "preventive care." This somehow has to be carried out for shots, dental care, eyes, and prescriptions.

- Why can't the government devise a simple way of obtaining the medical benefits for military retirees regardless of age? The first thing to do is consolidate the different programs into one. Example: let us abolish TRICARE, Extra TRICARE Standard, TRICARE Prime, Medicare, Medigap, TRICARE Senior, etc., and put them into one single program. A long time ago all we needed is a military ID card to be admitted into a hospital. Now we have so many ID cards that it is very confusing. There are so many different agencies, offices, telephone numbers, etc., not to mention the confusion of who, what, where to get the information just to get into a hospital. Just imagine how much money the government will save by eliminating those overlapping responsibilities in providing medical benefits to military retirees. JUST ONE ID card is what is really NEEDED!

- Currently I am in Secure Horizons. I may change to Kaiser. My physician retired. The local hospital is now an HCA facility. It's not so good. I hope the government takes care of the vets and their families who need help.

- Spouse is legally blind, no patience, [dislike] paperwork, [no] choice of doctors, hospital, etc. Haven't seen anything on costs, etc. Neither one of us drives—no car.

- Should one ask for a complete physical examination yearly? Many military [retirees] have asked me the above question. I notice people in their sixties and above are taking care of their health with little complaints.

- I am a retired veteran [and] professional engineer. Veteran Affairs [is] a gigantic mishmash of governmental meddling . . . an extravaganza with taxpayers' money—yet obviously failing . . . [with] strong-arm abuses of veterans. Medical performance follows "big-business" trends . . . no originality, no initiative. . . . System [is] frustrating for patients/veterans, equally for doctors. . . . Clinic appointment: No value received. Nothing learned, no doctor's counsel, no guidance. A photocopy of a five-year experience is attached. Perhaps it can be helpful. RAND questions required time and effort—was well spent to be helpful. Will *RAND reciprocate* with a *synopsis* of conclusions for Congress? . . . Reciprocation has been meager for diligent veterans. . . . Sad!

- Allow military retires and their family members to retain TRICARE when they become 65 years old. The 65-year-old military retires and their families should be eligible for TRICARE regardless if they are enrolled in Medicare Part B or the Federal Employees Health Plan. The National Defense Authorization Act (S.2549) should allow 65-year-olds in TRICARE if they are enrolled in the federal employees' health plan.

- We like to be able to decide what doctors we see and when we want to see them. Too many friends jumped into HMOs and are very unhappy now. They thought it would be cheaper and great. We are willing to pay to remain totally independent in our medical care. We have received no help from the military in the last 14 years except the military pharmacy and mail order under the BRAC program.

- It's hard to live a normal life on the money you get. Prices continue to go up and sometimes you go without medicine.

- We are both getting older and with age are not getting better.

- At the present time, have to drive too far for the hospital treatment.

- Hospital costs are high. I had outpatient surgery and the hospital bill alone was over $5,XXX. Fortunately my civilian job insurance paid costs after Medicare. I was at the hospital less than four hours. My prescription bill is around $4,XXX.00 per year. I answered questions as if I depended on military care—which I do not.

- No comments. We look forward to getting our drugs and medical care. Thanks.

- My spouse and I became eligible for TRICARE prescriptions April 1 and will be eligible for medical care under TRICARE with Medicare Part B, which we have at present.

- We live over 1XX miles from the closest military facility. In 199X I was diagnosed with [medical condition]. I did not want to change my coverage in the middle of the treatment.

- I went to the VA to have my disability increased. The VA did not increase it. I believe that the VA has an instruction NOT TO INCREASE DISABILITY [ratings or levels].

- Do not like having a doctor chosen for us. [Allow] the right and freedom of choosing our own doctor. Find that most doctors chosen in plans are not first class and some are not even [sector] physicians.

- Our government gives millions to other countries while many native U.S. citizens are homeless and have no medical care. Many had previous jobs, paid income tax, [paid for] Social Security and Medicare. [I blame it on] "downsizing" and U.S. companies moving to other countries.

- Need spouse to be a user of VA facilities. At present she is not eligible. I believe she should have the same coverage as I have.

Comments from Eligibles: Pharmacy Benefits

- In the last few years, prescriptions have taken a huge part of our income due to the fact that military pharmacies do not carry the drugs necessary, especially the newer drugs. Another need is dental and eye care.

- When I joined the Navy, I was told I and my dependents would have free medical and dental for life if I stayed for 20 years. It really irks me to have to pay anything for medical/dental. The new senior pharmacy national mail order program seemed that it was going to save us over $1,000 a year, but because we have a Medicare HMO with a pharmacy benefit I'm told we can't use it. On the other hand, if we had a military pharmacy convenient to us, we could take our prescriptions there and get them filled/refilled free even though we have HMO benefits—that's an inequity. I have recently become aware of another inequity in the pharmacy program. If you are an HMO member with pharmacy benefits, you cannot participate in senior pharmacy mail order but you can use the MTF pharmacy to get free medications. This policy discriminates against those who don't live close to an MTF pharmacy. I have to pay approximately $1,XXX a year for medications through an HMO pharmacy since a lot of medications are not on the list.

- The TRICARE for Life pharmacy plan starting 4-1-01 should be the same for all retirees. The mail-in plan and the retail plan should be available to All and no restrictions concerning TRICARE being second payee. Let there be no "caps" on their prescriptions from an HMO and other plans that may have your Medicare Part B assigned to them.

- My wife has cancer. We are eligible for prescription service with DoD NMOP through Merck-Medco Rx services. In October when TRICARE is able to furnish the same service, I will switch over. I had TRICARE Prime until I reached 65 and I was happy with it.

- Greatly appreciate the continuation of prescription services for members at age 65 plus.

- Our largest out-of-pocket cost is for prescriptions. When the military Merck-Medco mail order program became available several years ago, this cost was reduced. Now that VA care has become available with prescriptions available at no cost, our only medical coverage problem has disappeared for all [intents and] purposes. Had TRICARE coverage been available when I shifted to Medicare (5 years ago) we both would probably have enrolled.

- We are very dissatisfied with the prescription medication coverage by our current private health plans and fully support efforts by the military to care for its people, active or retired.

- Many of us live in small towns where the relationship with one doctor is often more than [just] patient-doctor. All things considered, I think the greatest benefit of TRICARE is prescription drugs. For people who have chronic illnesses (diabetes, high blood pressure, a hearing condition, etc.) the costs can be impossible to bear, whereas hospital and doctor's fees can be paid on installments, or sometime written off by the doctor or hospital. My biggest concern: Will this be permanent?

- At our age I feel it most important that we stay with a doctor that knows our history, the sickness we have, and has our records, which are extensive. Also it is important that we do not have to do a lot of traveling to get to a doctor (often twice a week.) The above is important but I feel that the cost of drugs is more important.

- Military pharmacy formularies change hourly. [The nearest military pharmacy is] 1XX miles away. The military doesn't want retirees and places conditions to exclude you. We have private insurance, a drug program with a copay, $20 and $40 dollars. The TRICARE drug program would not be a benefit in conjunction with [our] private insurance drug program. The military or government health program[s] tend [to be on a trial or temporary basis] or can be dropped without notice. [They are] not dependable. At our age, private insurance and Medicare is much more dependable. One cannot afford to abandon these programs for a temporary or trial basis. Drug program would be beneficial if copay was considered. TRICARE tends to be discriminatory for those who have private insurance.

- Your military pharmacy needs to carry more varieties of the same type of medications. Some people have side effects to some medications and your pharmacy does not carry the type that I can take without the side effects. I, the spouse, was not aware until this questionnaire that TRICARE was only a "demonstration" program.

- [For] some months we are unable to travel due to health to pick up prescriptions; therefore, we have to pay for them here. We also are on medication that our doctor does not want generically dispensed. My wife has allergies to numerous medications. We understood from information received that retirees were not entitled to TRICARE.

- We are not involved in the TRICARE Senior Supplement Demonstration Program. We are interested in some relief for prescription drugs. We are not close to a military base pharmacy; therefore, I must pay for our medications.

- My spouse utilizes the military pharmacy for her prescription drugs, however they do not stock some of the most expensive ones. These we purchase at the local civilian pharmacy at approximately $3XX per month.

- It greatly concerns me that all medications cost more almost at each refill. With a limited income the concern grows.

- Why are retirees not in a catchment area not covered for commercial pharmacies like those living where [there has been a] base closure?

- The benefits I receive from military pharmacies have been a great help.

Comments from Eligibles: "The Promise"

- All during my military career, we were told that as retirees we could continue to receive all military benefits we had received while on active duty. [This] included medical, dental, use of base facilities, etc., etc. Then Congress found out how much all that would cost, and began to restrict and reduce those benefits. All that remains is Medicare, which most civilians have. As WWII, Korea, Vietnam, and the Cold War receded from Congress's limited memories, many congressmen became disinterested, even anti-military. Such funded programs reduced the amount of "pork barrel" funds available to help with their reelection campaigns. Also, "special interest" funding became much more important to most, if not all, congressmen (and women). In short, military retirees are now treated as being in the same category as bastards were in the 18th century (as if we are nonexistent.) Commercial retailers through Congress forced base exchanges and commissaries [to the point that] retail costs to retirees equal or exceed costs at civilian retail stores. Retirees [are] paying the salaries of all those bureaucrats.

- Based on government actions over the past decade-plus, I have no military facilities remaining. All support promises made have been broken. I have no confidence in current or projected promises. I will watch for Action and then only over time. I will be looking for a History of positive action and only then ever trust again.

- Only information received on TRICARE is from military newsletter received in the mail. Not close to a military base.

- Based on "TRICARE for Life" and recent court rulings regarding the promise of free care, why are you wasting your time? I spent 2X years on active duty from 194X-197X and DoD is still doing trials! After retirement I spent 1X years working for [public employer] and have full coverage—dental, etc. They even pay my Medicare Part B.

- When I first enlisted in the USMC, I was told I would have free medical care for life at retirement (195X). My government has failed to live up to that promise.

- When I joined the Navy in 194X, I was promised free medical coverage for my spouse and I for life, provided I remain in the military until retirement. Today in 2001, all military facilities in my area have been closed.

- Before I was 65, military facilities were not available due to shortage of doctors, etc. After 65, I was told I was not eligible to use military facilities. I am waiting. Hopefully I will receive the benefits promised after serving 2X years of active military service.

- Due to the actions of the Congress in the past concerning health care from the military for retired personnel, I am not inclined to change my present status. The Congress of the United States cannot be depended upon for a long-term health plan for retired military personnel.

- The Navy promised to take care of me when I retired, then Congress (Congress, yeah) decided to close Oak Knoll Naval Hospital, then closed NAS, Moffett Field. Well, the HMO has done me pretty well, so guess I shouldn't complain.

- I hope this survey will help the many thousands of military retirees, and their families. As a military retiree, I was promised health care for the rest of my life if I made the military service my career. When I reached 62, my I.D. Card was changed and disallowed me and my spouse to use military hospital facilities. I was very bitter. However, now I have hope that the government will fulfill its promise to all military retirees. Thank You Very Much.

- Was in the U.S. Navy for 2X years and was always informed when I re-enlisted, and even after I was retired for many years, the military got free health insurance for the rest of our lives. This was not true and is still not true. I will never pay for health insurance that the military and my U.S.A. government promised. I'm sure that I will die and not get what I was promised, so I do not believe most of what the military and the political people in my country, U.S.A, tell us. What a shame. Join the military and you can become cannon fodder for the rich. They do not care and never have.

- I enlisted in 194X, and retired in 196X. For that entire period, I was promised free medical and dental care for life. As late as 1991, these promises were still being made. These promises were in writing. Congress has taken care of themselves with FEHBP—the Federal Employees Health Benefit Plan which did NOT cover the military. Isn't it about time that the promises made are kept? Your survey asks the wrong questions. Your questions are slanted to make people think they must pay for medical care even though they were promised free medical and dental care. You should be asking why people think they are not getting what was promised.

- At the time of my enlistment in 194X, I was told that the government would provide free lifetime medical treatment after 20 years of service, and this was inferred at reenlistment times. I am fortunate to have the Federal Employees Health Benefit! I [was covered] through my employment with the [federal government] and I joined an HMO (Kaiser) after retirement from there. My medical and Kaiser medical insurance runs approximately $2,000.00 a year plus another two to three hundred in copayments from doctor visits and prescriptions.

- It was fortunate that I worked after military retirement to get medical care for me and my family. The military has not been there for many years.

- This has been very hard for me do, for when I was a young man, the government told me if I stayed in the military for 20 years, myself and my spouse would be taken care of medically in all forms "pertaining" to our "health" for the rest of our lives. I was told a few years ago at a military or VA hospital, "They lied to you and there is nothing you can do about it." I'm extremely disappointed in the fact that thousands of Americans were led to believe that "if" they took care of their country, their country would take of them! Thank you.

- Military retirees were promised free medical care. All local military treatment facilities including secondary or specialty areas have been closed down. My nearest MTF is Trans AFB, more than 1XX miles from my home. DoD owes us veterans, especially those of us who served in WWII and other conflicts and remained in the service, to make good on that promise.

- I was told at VA that the so-called "TRICARE" will not be available until October! My wife doesn't have any medical coverage aside from Medicare A and B, and Kaiser's Senior Advantage coverage. This worried me because it's more than I can afford! Senior Advantage costs $30 a month. When I choose a military career, I thought my wife would also be covered by the same medical coverage as mine! Another unfulfilled promise!

- I was under the impression I would have free medical care the rest of my life once I retired from the Navy as I was promised—What happened?!!!

- I am a retired military officer [who served in] WWII and the Korean War—2X years total service. My military retirement medical benefits are worthless to me! And to my wife!

- The government should keep their promises to the military retirees to give us medical [benefits] throughout our life.

- We do not have much information on our TRICARE for Life yet but it looks as though we are on the right track. Since our military service began during a time when health care was promised for life, then so be it—that is the way it should be.

- I am not satisfied with the cost of various care plans now offered retirees and their dependents. When I entered the army in 193X, the government stated, in writing, that retirees would be provided free medical care and prescription service for life. This also applied to legal dependents of retirees. I served for 2X years—including service in WWII and occupation duty in Germany. Why can't the U.S. government keep its promises to retirees?

- I was told for 20 years that military medical care would be available to me and my family for life. Have not had access to same for 17 years.

- Enrolled on a "why not?" basis as a backup in case my Medigap HMO defaults. I am an M.D. (retired) and while not rich, in comfortable circumstances. Therefore, I am far from typical. As an M.D., I feel most military retirees are NOT getting what they were promised!

- I enlisted in the Navy in 194X and stayed in until 196X. Mostly I kept shipping over as each enlistment ended because I believed the Navy when they said, "Sign right here, son, and we will take care of all your health needs, forever." On top of that, they finally yanked the rug out from under the many retired military here in the San Francisco Bay Area by closing down the only Navy hospital. Now I'm with Secure Horizons, who used to be okay but now their membership payments keep escalating outrageously.

- When I joined the Navy in 194X, I was guaranteed full medical coverage upon retirement. With the cutback of military bases, I would like to use VA hospitals if TRICARE becomes a permanent system for senior retirees.

- When I was serving in the uniform of our nation, I was promised that I would receive military medical care for the rest of my life. [We were promised] medical care to retirees at less cost to taxpayers and our own choice of doctor.

- What happened to the FREE medical care promised? The experimental program will still require a supplement to cover costs Medicare doesn't authorize. No one knows what is covered until you get a bill! Information

I've received indicates the program hasn't started until April or October?? The BRAC pharmacy program is SUPER! I wonder how long it will last. We retired vets get promises—they usually fall through the budget cracks!

- I am WWII vet. The government promised me and my deceased wife free medical care for life if I served for 20 years for my country. I served for 3X years. I deserve better.

- I think that the government has let all retirees down by not providing free healthcare as stated as an incentive to remain on active duty. This TRICARE does not meet my needs and is too expensive. The dental is also more expensive than it should be for a government program. How can the government fail those of us who gave our service during WWII and continued through retirement?

- My biggest expense ever—for medical problems—was last year. [It was] $XX00.00 for dental work, and I expect to spend the same amount again as soon as I can get a hold of it. The military did a . . . poor job of dental work on me during the 2X years I spent in the military. All in all, military health is adequate, and more than most [who are] not in the military get. Thanks for this. Strange, though, that now that I have been retired for "40" years they "might" be going to do something that they contracted to do a long, long time ago. It probably will not help me, but maybe someone else.

- I have been most fortunate in having good health coverage from my employer. I know that other retirees from military service are less fortunate than I. When I entered the service in 195X we were told we would have the same things that retired duty personnel have. This unfortunately has not been true.

- I believe the U.S. military should keep their promises to retired servicemen for FREE lifetime medical and dental coverage for themselves and their dependents, which includes hospitalization, prescriptions, preventive care, and office visits. But with the closing of so many military facilities, a possible solution is for the military (DoD) to [give] support with construction maintenance, staffing, and monetary assistance for retired military veterans and their dependents to use the Veterans Administration Medical Centers and facilities on a free No Cost basis.

- I was promised lifetime medical care for free for myself and my dependents if I served a minimum of twenty years on active duty. The U.S. government has broken their promise. This promise was the main reason I chose to make the Navy a career. The Department of Defense should reinstate this lifetime medical treatment and apologize for their [mistreatment].

- We were told we would, for the rest of our lives (including our spouses' lives), receive free medical treatment through the military. Then to have that treatment stop when we reached age 65 (it is from that age on when we need more care), it is more than a breach of a contract. It is an immoral act that needs correcting! (Such an agreement may not have been in writing, but it certainly was an oral contract each time I re-up'd over the 20 years I devoted my youth serving in the military, and expected the nation to stand by its oral commitments/contracts.)

- Don't know anything about TRICARE. To live up to promises made by the government for retirees, they need to have a CHAMPUS-style policy as a second insurance for Medicare.

- To Whom It May Concern: I am a Navy veteran of 3X years, retiring an HTCS from the U.S. Navy. After retiring from the Navy 2X years ago, I have not used any of my medical benefits at military hospitals or facilities. Now upon reaching Social Security age, my health is not as good as years gone by. I now need more medical benefits and prescription drugs at low cost. I cannot afford high-price prescriptions for myself and my wife. Upon reaching 65, I could no longer use CHAMPUS. All my medical was taken away. Then [when] I did try to use a military hospital or facility, I was turned away. The closest base to me is 1XX miles away. It is in Shreveport, Louisiana, or Fort Polk, Louisiana. I live in Texas. I was promised medical benefits for the rest of my life and [for my] dependents. The U.S. took all that away. I think it is about time the U.S. government got behind its military. I need, and so do the other veterans who served their county and served it proudly, low-cost medical and prescriptions. We need the option to choose our own doctors and hospitals. Before reaching 65 years of age, it was such a hassle using CHAMPUS. All the paperwork and then being turned down was quite a headache. You could never get through to their lines. Always busy and very frustrating. Let us hope that the U.S.A. stands behind its veterans and gives them back what [they were promised when] they proudly fought for the country. Give us what was promised to us—our medical and our prescriptions without any hassle and at low cost.

- I served for 3X years and was promised that I would have free medical care for life.

- When me and my wife retired from the military we chose a town close to a military base for the benefits that were promised and then the benefits finally just went away.

- 1. My government promised me total health care for life when I entered in 195X. 2. If properly designed, TRICARE for Life fulfills that promise. 3. Pharmacy privileges/access are a must.

- [It is] over 1XX miles to the nearest care [facility]. With the limit on appointments, you could not get both at Barksdale AFB. The service promised me medical care for life at age 65 and they reneged on the promise. As a recruiter, I promised hundreds the same thing. This makes me out to be a liar also. I would not be ashamed or against signing [up for the program].

- I put in 20+ years of service to my country! We were guaranteed health care the rest of our lives. Why are you always trying to jam something less down our throats? We want what we were promised when I joined the service in 195X. The VA takes good care of me 100%. My spouse is not 65 yet, so what can you offer us? We need CHAMPUS or something like that [type of health care]. [My wife] has a supplement until she gets to be 65 then she will have Medicare and we will change her supplement to support Medicare. Need help for [the next] 3 years.

- When I enlisted, the recruiters told me that I would have free medical for the rest of my life if I made a career of the military. I also recruited under the same policy of free medical under guidelines set by the 9th Naval District. This period was from 196X–196X in [state]. No mention of any other CHAMPUS supplements to health care was ever told to me.

- I had [medical treatment]. Because of the loss of my military benefits, I would not have been able to have these treatments if it were not for the fact the VA took care of it for me. Our government outright lied to all of us military retirees. Therefore, I have lost all respect for our government. I doubt I'll ever regain that respect. The government does not deserve our respect or loyalty.

- As a military retiree, I feel that full medical and dental was promised to me for 20-plus years as an inducement to reenlist, only to see these promises broken one by one from 196X until present. Not only were these benefits promised to me, but also for my spouse and dependent children. YES, IT'S ABOUT TIME.

- At the time I decided to make the service a career I was led to believe that I would have free military-sponsored medical care for the rest of my life for myself and my family. This has proved to not be true.

- Long years ago, I was promised by the government I would have health care for life. Baloney.

- Why doesn't the military take care of retirees as I was told they would, or provide free medical care or all that Medicare does not?

- Due to my being promised free medical care all this time throughout my long military life, I think the government has reneged on its promise to me.

- We were never offered TRICARE because as we understood from people at the Barksdale base we were not in an area where it was offered. I think that my country has let me down since I turned 65, that they said, we don't need you anymore because you can't be on standby for recall to active duty to help us in need.

- It is gratifying to know that our nation has made official its decades-old promise of lifetime health care for military members who accept the unique demands and sacrifices inherent in a career in uniform.

- When I enlisted in 195X I was promised health care if I stayed for 20 years. I stayed and served with honor—my country failed to keep its promise. I have spent $30,000 on health care and insurance since becoming 65 years old that I shouldn't have had to.

- During my 3X years active duty service in the U.S. Navy, I was promised full medical care (at no cost to me) for myself and eligible dependents. For 3X years I was lied to. Even though my pay was very low for many of my 3X years, and tours of duty were far from safe or enjoyable at times, I still looked forward to having my family and my medical needs met (at no out-of-pocket costs) as promised. This promise of "no-cost medical care" was one of the most important reasons myself and thousands of others decided, without hesitation, to pursue a career in the United States Armed Forces.

- When I entered the service (I spent 20+ years) I was told if I stayed for 20 years my medical would be paid for life.

- I believe it is the responsibility of the military to provide health and prescription drugs to military retires. That was the commitment I was given to understand when I entered the military in 194X.

- During my military career, I was promised health care for life. After retirement it almost disappeared and after reaching 65 it did disappear. My insurance was great, so I elected not to take Medicare Part B when I became 65. Then I learned that by law my insurance could only pay what Part B would pay. Now to participate in the TRICARE program, I must take Part B and pay a penalty for the rest of my life. Is there something wrong with this picture? I think everything is wrong with this picture.

- Military retirees were deceived about their medical benefits during their years of active duty. They should have supplemental insurance at no cost to them or should have CHAMPUS as needed!

- [I had a medical procedure] three years ago. Had to pay out of pocket what Medicare did not pay [because I had] no insurance. The VA would not see me since I retired with nothing wrong, said I made too much money. The VA is a big joke to people like me. I have to go to an active duty military base to get my prescriptions filled. Had [where I worked] insurance and CHAMPUS till age 65 then was put on Medicare. Cannot afford to buy insurance now. Most insurance won't take you if you have [medical conditions]. The U.S.A. needs to take care of vets at no cost. We gave up higher salaries for military service, did [not] save much in service or accumulate much. Was told at the Army base in Ft. Polk that I did not live in a TRICARE area. So, [the government] takes our taxes and sends them everywhere but where some of us need it. If I sound bitter, I am.

- Military retirees were promised health care for the rest of their lives.

- Our congressmen and senators need to give more consideration to our veterans. I know we have a few "professional veterans" who knock military medical service and VA services. Overall it is good. Let's improve it and take care of our military retirees [and see they get] good care.

- When I enlisted in the service (195X) I was promised medical care for life for myself as well as my family. This has not happened because of politicians taking it away from me and all were told the same thing. It is a shame that the government has abandoned all the men and women that gave their all for this same government. Totally free medical should be restored to all retirees and their families.

- I think it is a shame and a disgrace that military retirees and spouses don't get the free medical coverage that was promised to them when they enlisted into the military. I retired with 2X years of service and I am not eligible for VA hospital care as I was told when I tried to sign up. I'll bet that there is not a congressman or senator that is not eligible for government health benefits (yes, I am very bitter).

- We gave our life to the military and were promised lifetime care. A bill has been passed, but it should not be a "burden" to get care under it. The HMOs have not worked. If this is tailored after HMOs, it won't work either.

- We were promised that if we served our country over 20 years, our medical care for ourselves and our family, including our children through the age of eighteen, would be taken care of. This was an outright lie by our government. I have been out tens of thousands of dollars for insurance and prescription drugs since my retirement. A class action lawsuit should be filed against Congress and the federal government for their lies and deceit. I am a disabled veteran. I don't trust the VA hospitals because I think they're second-rate. I have no problem with paying for a deductible to pay for administration expenses. Thank you for your concern.

- I was promised health [care] for life at no cost.

- I retired from the U.S. Navy in 197X (2X years of service). I was promised free medical care for life for me and my spouse. U.S. government reneged on their promise!

- I along with thousands of vets believe that our hospitalization should be provided by the government we so proudly served as they had said they would do.

- Provide lifetime medical care as promised throughout my low-paying career; medical services at least equal to that provided a retired U.S. federal worker.

- When I first enlisted (194X) I was promised health care for life if I stayed in at least 20 years. My government did not keep their promise. My wife and I did what was necessary, to assume at least a reasonable level of health care when we retired. Many of my shipmates have not been as fortunate for one reason or another. This plan will help make amends. This said, I think it's an excellent health plan, especially the drug options. Thank You.

- The CHAMPUS/TRICARE Plan should be abolished! Those Bureaucratic Personnel who concocted the TRICARE Plan should be institutionalized for proper mental care. All retired military personnel and their legal dependants should receive "free" medical care, including pharmaceuticals anytime, anywhere upon presentation of a valid military identification card. Validity of the card should be checked via the computer network. The same should apply to all personnel on active duty. There must not be any restrictions placed on the service. Currently, I am under Medicare. We all know that this system is a failure and requires supplemental insurance to keep the recipient out of bankruptcy. But in many cases the insurance payments, co-payments, deductibles, and pharmaceuticals will still generate bankruptcy. Should the spouse of the recipient not be under Medicare, then bankruptcy is assured. The medication my spouse is on is constantly being changed; therefore, a DoD mail order pharmacy will not suffice. Military pharmacies have been drastically cut back and cannot fill the prescriptions required. The closest facility is 1XX miles from my home. TRICARE Senior Supplement Demonstration Program! I do not know what this program is but it appears to be another bureaucratic scheme dreamed up by a group of "bubbleheads" to evade the government's responsibilities related to free health care to military retirees and their dependents. Should we be prepared to bend over for this program? I am much more interested in proper medical care for my dependants than for myself. Without their suffering and full support, I and many others would not now be a military retiree.

- If I had failed in my duties and responsibilities while on active duty as the DoD has done toward my family and me in retirement, I would have been C.M. [court-martialed]. My word, deeds, and actions had to be above board. I could not turn my back on promised responsibility as the DoD did since 1966.

- It is about time.

- The military health care is not dependable; it changes with the wind. Private industry and civil service federal benefits are superior to the military benefits. Military retirees have been left out and lied to constantly. The old saying has proven true, i.e., during wartime (declared war) nothing is too good for the military and nothing is what they get in peacetime or when retired. Vagrants on the streets are more important to the federal government than retired military!

- I was promised free medical care for me and my spouse upon completion of 20 years service. I met my part of the bargain. Any program that requires a fee or copay for prescriptions is a slap in the face by the government of the country I dedicated my life to for over 20 years.

- Any out-of-pocket expense is a violation of the military contract of lifetime free medical care for myself and my spouse and even TFL does not answer this promise!

- The coverage is only available for a limited period of time. Would not want to drop a private insurance plan and accept TRICARE when the plan may not last. The government promised years ago that military retirees would be provided with health care. This has not happened. Who can say it will be provided in the future?

- About 3 years ago, Barksdale AFB, Louisiana, told us to leave because we lived more than 40 miles from the base and could not use their facilities. So I'm thinking of transferring my family service records to Fort Polk, Louisiana. On a scale of 1-10, this base is a 2—Bad. About 2 years ago, we were traveling and tried to fill a prescription at Tinder AFB, Oklahoma. Those people met us at the door and really treated us nice. On a scale of 1–10, I give Tinker AFB a 12. I really don't care who knows, I would tell Congress the same thing.

- Since I've been on Social Security, I have been paying premiums on Medicare A and B, which I have not used. I was promised, as a military retiree, free medical care for my family and me for life. I truly believed what I was promised. I am grateful for the medical attention I do get from the VA, both the clinic and the hospital, and I am a little miffed, but not upset, that I pay a small fee for my medication. They are overworked and crowded, but the VA is doing a good job on limited resources. My wife, of course, receives no VA help, and her expenses are increasing every year. Thank you.

- I entered military service in 195X. I and my peers were promised health care for life if we stayed until retirement (20 years). This promise was given verbally in earlier years and written in agreement later on. Nevertheless, I believe it to be morally binding. For the last 25 years, I have paid enormous premiums for supplemental insurance for my wife and me. It is time for a generous change.

Comments from Eligibles: Provider Access

- [My] current care is with Palo Alto medical foundation. When considering TRICARE trial, I was told by them "we do not accept TRICARE." I could not leave my specialist so did not enroll [in TRICARE]. I will certainly enroll this fall.

- There [was] no military medical facility [after] bases were closed. [We] should be able to go any doctor we choose.

- Did not feel hospitals and doctors in this area were familiar enough concerning the TRICARE program. Thank you for the privilege of voicing my opinion on this matter.

- We both receive complete health care at no cost.

- My wife's provider will not accept TRICARE. Reasons: low pay, slow pay. She needs a doctor regularly who will accept TRICARE. Her doctor accepts AARP and Medicare so we must stay with [those plans]. I have never received an application to join TRICARE. And have never received instructions on how to enroll.

- The area we live in is *not* committed to helping military retirees. A hospital is under construction but as of [date] no one is willing to say, "Yes, we will accept TRICARE." TRICARE is not accepted now in the local hospital.

- A lot of doctors will not accept TRICARE because they are not paid enough.

- My spouse is on TRICARE Standard, which she has a lot of trouble [with] because the doctors will not except TRICARE. Because it pays so little they said they can not except it. We live in a small town and the nearest military base is [7X] miles [away].

- Many doctors and hospitals and pharmacies complained that TRICARE took way too long to respond and way too long to pay the providers. As a result, some won't contract with them.

G. Maps of Demonstration Areas

The TRICARE Senior Supplement Demonstration, scheduled to end on December 31, 2002, was conducted in and around Santa Clara County, California, and Cherokee County, Texas. Eligible beneficiaries must have resided in a defined area surrounding these locations and be a retiree of the Uniformed Services, a dependent of a Uniformed Services retiree, or the dependent survivor of a Uniformed Services retiree or member.

The maps on the following pages of this appendix illustrate the location of the TSSD enrollees at each demonstration site.

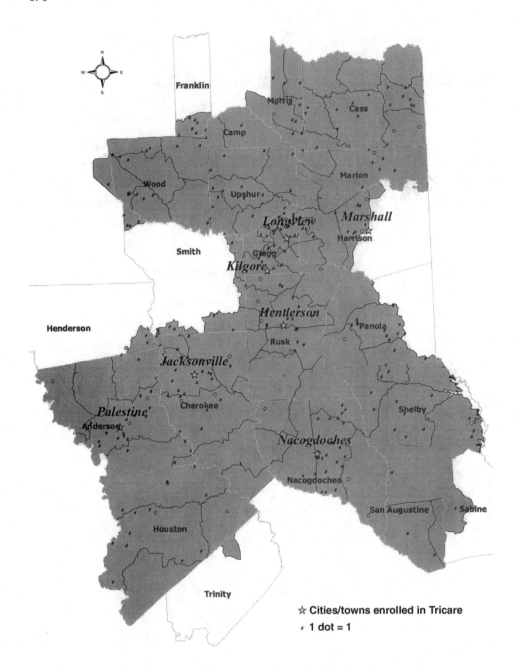

Figure G.1—TSSD Enrollees in and Around Cherokee County, Texas

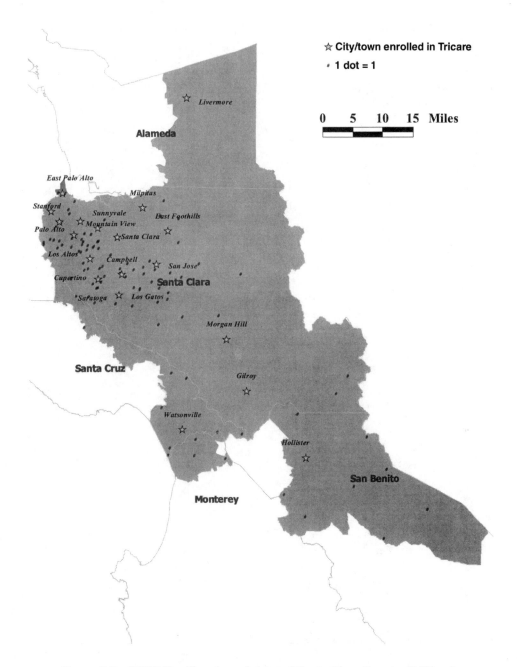

Figure G.2—TSSD Enrollees in and Around Santa Clara County, California

References

Cecchine G., K. M. Harris, A. Suarez, and M. Schoenbaum, "TRICARE Senior Supplement Demonstration Evaluation Focus Group Results," Santa Monica, Calif., unpublished RAND research.

Department of Defense/TRICARE Management Activity, *The TRICARE Senior Supplement Demonstration Program: Extending Your Health Care Benefits*, n.d., www.tricare.osd.mil/tssd.

Department of Veterans Affairs, *VA Long Term Care at the Cross Roads: Report of the Federal Advisory Committee on the Future of VA Long-Term Care*, Washington, D.C., June 1998.

Farley, D. O., K. M. Harris, J. S. Ashwood, G. J. Dydek, and J. B. Carleton, *The First Year of the Medicare-DoD Subvention Demonstration: Evaluation Report for FY99*, Santa Monica, Calif.: RAND, MR-1271.0-HCFA, 2000.

Goodno, D., TMA administrator for TSSD, e-mail correspondence, November 14, 2000.

Health Care Financing Administration, data on the general Medicare population for March 2000, http://www.hcfa.gov/medicare/mgd-rept.htm.

Medicare, summary information on the benefits of the Ten Standardized Medigap plans, http://www.medicare.gov/mgcompare/Search/StandardizedPlans/TenStandardPlans.asp.

Public Law 89-614, Military Medical Benefits Amendments of 1966.

Schoenbaum, M., K. M. Harris, G. Cecchine, M. Bradley, A. Suarez, T. Tanielian, and C. R. Anthony, *Final Evaluation Report for Uniformed Services Continuous Open Enrollment Demonstration*, Santa Monica, Calif.: RAND, MR-1352-OSD, 2001.

Sturm, R., J. Unutzer, and W. Katon, "Effectiveness Research and Implications for Study Design: Sample Size and Statistical Power, *Gen Hosp Psychiatry*, Vol. 21, No. 4, 1999, pp. 274–283.

TRICARE Management Activity, information on TRICARE Plus, http://www.tricare.osd.mil/Plus/default.htm.

Urban Institute Analyses of 1997 Medicare Current Beneficiary Survey, cited in *Medicare at a Glance*, Henry J. Kaiser Family Foundation, Menlo Park, Calif., June 2001.

U.S. General Accounting Office, *Defense Health Care: Tri-Service Strategy Needed to Justify Medical Resources for Readiness and Peacetime Care*, GAO/HEHS-00-10, November 1999.